# STUFF YOU SHOULD KNOW ABOUT

# RHEUMATOID ARTHRITIS

## DR IRWIN LIM

ISBN: 978-1-925590-51-7 (first edition)
Published by Vivid Publishing
A division of Fontaine Publishing Group
P.O. Box 948, Fremantle
Western Australia 6959
www.vividpublishing.com.au

Cataloguing-in-Publication data is available from the National Library of Australia

# Contents

# About me (and BJC Health)

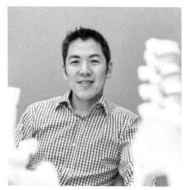

As a rheumatologist, my job involves diagnosing and treating all sorts of diseases affecting muscles, bones, tendons, and joints. There's detective work, with explanation and education, followed by formulation of a plan of action to try and improve the situation when this is possible.

My other role is as a director of BJC Health. BJC Health is a dynamic, multidisciplinary group clinic which focuses on providing comprehensive, coordinated treatment solutions for people suffering with arthritis & related diseases.

I am heavily involved in the clinic's educational activities for allied health professionals and GPs and I strongly believe in the need for patient education, empowerment and engagement.

Now working through my 5th decade on this planet, I do try to improve my own health while I try to integrate my busy, fulfilling work life with the roles of husband and father to three school-aged children.

# Dedication

I have to dedicate this book to my wife, Mary. She's patiently read every post I've written, and provided me the indulgence of time, time spent on Facebook, twitter, LinkedIn and my blog. While she rightfully teaches our kids to be wary of strangers on the internet and to be wary about what they expose about themselves, she seems to have turned a blind eye on my exploits. Then again, she does seem to track and read a lot of the stuff I am posting…

# Introduction

I started using social media to educate at the end of 2010. I was never sure how long I would continue but it's become something that I'm unlikely to stop.

A clear benefit for me has been a much greater awareness of what those who have chronic arthritis, such as rheumatoid arthritis, experience. Uncertainty, frustration, various side effects, misunderstanding, and also importantly, hope.

It's easy enough, and I have done this myself, to suggest that those people (doctors prefer the term patients), who use social media to discuss their problems, must be those who are not doing well or those who are "difficult", needing somewhere to vent their frustrations.

Those people with rheumatoid arthritis who are doing well aren't exactly spending a lot of time telling others how well they do. They just get on with their lives, don't they?

I think there is truth in this. But there is a clear space and need for better communication, for people to learn more about their disease, for them to have resources to point their friends and family to, those people who are struggling to understand.

At the start of the journey, people do search for information. They may not actively engage in discussion but they're reading and learning.

Unfortunately, most rheumatologists confine their contribution to patient education to the consultation rooms.

So people with rheumatoid arthritis upon searching online will often come across blogs from other people with rheumatoid arthritis who for whatever reason have decided to share their experience or to work as an advocate.

These are really useful. I do however feel that a physician's voice is needed.

I've written many posts over the years dealing with rheumatoid arthritis. With this book, I've decided to collate these, and to flesh out some of these thoughts.

It's not meant to be an authoritative textbook or a manual to explain every single symptom or every single possible side effect various medications may have. It certainly doesn't replace the research I hope you'd be doing about this disease.

Rather, I see it as a starting point.

A resource to help you understand what your rheumatology team is thinking. And perhaps, one that will better help you appreciate aspects of rheumatoid arthritis so you can have better conversations about your management with family, friends and your health support team.

# Structure of this book

I've chosen a number of blog posts written about rheumatoid arthritis between December 2010 and early 2017 which remain relevant.

These have been rearranged into a structure that hopefully makes sense.

Where possible, I've updated links and provided higher quality photos and pictures than those originally posted.

I have tried to correct obvious spelling and punctuation mistakes in the blog posts, without changing sentence structure or the actual content.

Many of the blog posts end with a question.

In the original web format, this attracted answers and comments from readers, many of whom also have chronic arthritis and rheumatoid arthritis. With some of the posts, I think you'll find these comments enriching so I've included the links to the webpages for you to peruse.

I've then added thoughts and explanations around these blog posts to help you better understand, or to introduce concepts and ideas that I've not actually previously written about.

# Chapter 1

When the term "arthritis" is used, many people think of a disease affecting older people. This is not true, especially for Rheumatoid Arthritis (RA).

RA affects young people as well. The peak incidence for the onset is thought to be between 30-50 years but it can occur at a wide range of ages.

Our immune system normally focuses on fighting bacteria and virus, but in RA, it gets it wrong becoming overaggressive. The immune system then directs the fight against parts of you.

## Rheumatoid Arthritis: What is it?
Published May 24, 2011

One of the major diseases we have expertise in treating in BJC Health is Rheumatoid Arthritis. I thought it was time to explain to you what RA is.

### RA is an autoimmune disease.

Normally, your body's immune system helps fight off infections, keeping you healthy. With an autoimmune disease, this very complex immune system becomes a little disordered, resulting in some healthy tissues in the body being attacked.

In rheumatoid arthritis, the immune system attacks the lining of the joints, a tissue called synovium. This leads to inflammation and joint damage.

While research into causes of rheumatoid arthritis are advanced, we still do not know the exact reason why the immune system does this.

### RA is common.

About 1% of the population is affected with this disease. Rheumatoid arthritis tends to run in families. It is more common in women, occurring twice or thrice as frequently as it does in men. Smoking clearly increases the risk of developing rheumatoid arthritis, and leads to more severe disease.

### RA causes pain, stiffness & swelling of the joints.

Typically, the smaller joints, such as those in the hands and feet are affected earlier. However, larger joints such as the hips and knees are also often involved.

### RA causes suffering & loss of function.

In many patients, rheumatoid arthritis is a progressive illness that may cause joint destruction with reduction in a person's functional ability. This may mean difficulty with simple daily tasks such as gripping or dressing, or it may mean pain with walking. Simple activities we usually take for granted.

### RA requires early referral & treatment.

This is a disease that really benefits from early intervention. Early diagnosis followed by early, effective treatment prevents much of the joint destruction and deformity. As a result, early referral to a rheumatologist is crucial to avoid missing this period, known as the window of opportunity.

### Rheumatoid Arthritis is a serious disease.

It's not "just arthritis". There's a good chance you'll know someone with this problem & hopefully, this post will help you understand a little more about what they're going through.

# What causes RA?

Most patients will ask me what causes the disease. We don't really know. While the exact cause of RA has not been worked out, we have gained significant understanding of this disease at a molecular level over the last one to two decades.

By this, I mean that scientists have started to work out how your immune cells communicate and signal each other, and where this signalling goes astray in autoimmune disease. This has then led to better informed decisions about what medications and therapies to develop given their more likely success.

It's believed that certain environmental factors are required to switch on the defective immune pathway in a person who is genetically susceptible.

RA is clearly more common in smokers and there is evidence that smoking results in more aggressive disease. There are also emerging associations with periodontal disease and with lung infections.

## Rheumatoid Arthritis is...?
Published September 13, 2012

I was involved in an inservice for our BJC Health physiotherapists and exercise physiologists. Our team already know about rheumatoid arthritis but my brief was to discuss cases with them and to try and give them a deeper understanding into this common disease.

I decided to start with a simple challenge.

Pretend that I'm not a rheumatologist, but instead, a patient who has just been told their diagnosis.

How would you explain what rheumatoid arthritis is?

In terms that I can understand and comprehend.

I picked on Belinda first and then the others chimed in. The right words were mentioned. Autoimmune. Treat early. Effective treatment now exists. Inflammatory. Swollen and tender joints. Lots of stiffness. Deformity. Erosions.

They all knew stuff about rheumatoid arthritis. But, they weren't very good in putting it succinctly and in simple terms. This is of course, not surprising.

Rheumatoid arthritis is a complex disease. In fact, it's not just one disease but more a label that we typically apply to a certain set of symptoms and signs.

All rheumatologists would have a spiel that they adapt for the patient in front of them. The spiel is typically an oversimplification. By necessity, the complexities of the disease are purposely ignored (at that particular time).

Instead, the key messages need to be sold. The patient can then begin a process of education, to whatever level of complexity that they are comfortable with, and over time, the rheumatologist can then introduce the more complicated issues. If required.

I ask you to help me/us with this starting point. I am very interested to know how you readers (patients, rheumatologists, academics, BJC Staff, patient activists) would complete this:

"Rheumatoid Arthritis is ..."

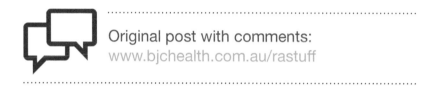

Original post with comments:
www.bjchealth.com.au/rastuff

# Chapter 2

## Signs + Symptoms

RA commonly affects the small joints of the hands and feet. It usually affects both sides and is said to occur in a roughly symmetrical pattern. A common scenario is for patients to describe swelling, pain, and stiffness associated with reduced handgrip power and function for a few hours in the morning.

Don't however get hung up about this if this is not your pattern. Early on, the disease may only be present on one side and even with time, it is not perfectly symmetrical.

In addition, the larger joints such as wrists, elbows, shoulders, hips, knees and ankles can be affected. Sometimes, the joint at the jaw, the temporomandibular joint is involved. RA can also affect the neck, in particular the first two segments of the cervical spine, presenting as upper neck pain.

The affected joints can be inflamed with some combination of swelling, heat and tenderness. Symptoms are typically worse at rest and early in the morning, and can improve with activity.

## Rheumatoid doesn't need to start with hand arthritis
Published March 30, 2016

My friend who is also a doctor missed her rheumatoid arthritis for some time.

It's been awhile since med school and she has the same idea about rheumatoid arthritis as so many others.

The picture she remembers involves hands with hand swelling, hand pain, hand arthritis and a degree of deformity.

Note that this does not need to be the case and deformity is clearly a VERY LATE presentation, and one we can and need to avoid.

She had many months of pain at the balls of the feet. She blamed this on needing to be on her feet a lot at work.

But, in retrospect, the symptoms were inflammatory in nature, with stiffness and a sensation of tightness first thing in the morning. And there was a degree of intermittent swelling.

Mild enough to ignore. Unfortunately.

As this is what most do. Understandably.

Ignore. Explain away. Get on with life.

When the symptoms finally started in her knuckles (her metacarpophalangeal joints), the penny dropped and she referred herself to a rheumatologist.

Rheumatoid Arthritis can start in many joints. The forefeet, typically at the metatarsophalangeal joints, is a common area.

But the initial joints involved could be a shoulder, the wrists, an elbow, the jaw region (temporomandibular joint), the neck, a knee, the ankles or midfeet.

The small joints of the hands are often involved at some stage, but the purpose of this post is to inform you that this doesn't always have to be the case.

Which joints did your rheumatoid arthritis start in?

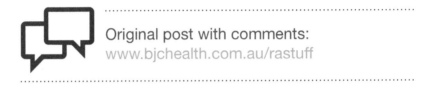

Original post with comments:
www.bjchealth.com.au/rastuff

Please note that RA is not confined to joints.

It can affect other organs in the body, so called extra-articular manifestations. A common problem is dryness of the eyes and mouth, but it can also result in inflammation of the lining of the heart and lungs (pericarditis and pleurisy) and scarring of the lungs (pulmonary fibrosis).

The clinical course of RA is generally one of exacerbations and remissions.

## 12 ways rheumatoid arthritis hurts you
Published May 30, 2011

Rheumatoid Arthritis is considered first & foremost a joint disease, an arthritis.

RA can start in any joint but most commonly, the smaller joints of the fingers & the wrists are affected. These smaller joints in the hands are the "knuckles": the metacarpophalangeal joints (MCPJs) and/or the proximal interphalangeal joints (PIPJs).

The pattern of involvement is described as symmetrical. This means that if 1 joint is swollen and painful on one hand, a similar joint is often (but not always) involved on the other hand.

However, like most of the autoimmune diseases, rheumatoid arthritis has wider, systemic effects.

It's not just a joint problem.

The disease itself can cause other symptoms, apart from
1)     joint pain, swelling & tenderness.

These include:

2)     Fatigue: can be debilitating & slow to improve

3)     Stiffness: noted mainly in the morning & after sitting for long periods

4)     A sensation of weakness

5)     Rheumatoid Nodules: lumps under the skin found on elbows & other bony surfaces

6)     Loss of appetite

7)     Muscle pain

8)     Depression

9) Dryness of the mouth & eyes: known as "sicca" or secondary Sjogren's syndrome

10) In more severe or in untreated disease, organ involvement: includes inflammatory eye disease such as scleritis, lung disease, and inflammation of blood vessels (rheumatoid vasculitis).

11) Increase in cardiovascular risks

12) Accelerated bone loss, with an increase in osteoporosis

Rheumatologists in general, understandably focus on the joint symptoms, as we know that by arresting joint erosion by early treatment (the window of opportunity), we can effectively prevent a lot of the joint deformity & destruction.

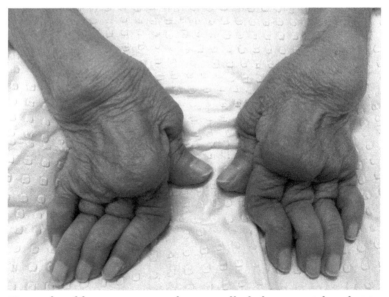

*Example of late stage, poorly controlled rheumatoid arthritis. This is what we need to prevent.*

However, sufferers with rheumatoid arthritis often continue to have some of the symptoms listed above even after the joint disease is seemingly controlled.

A comprehensive, multidisciplinary, coordinated approach to the management of this disease would appear to be a good thing. BJC Health continues to develop a Connected Care approach to rheumatoid arthritis.

If you have rheumatoid arthritis, do you suffer with some of the listed symptoms?

Apart from medication, what are other components of your current management plan?

Original post with comments:
www.bjchealth.com.au/rastuff

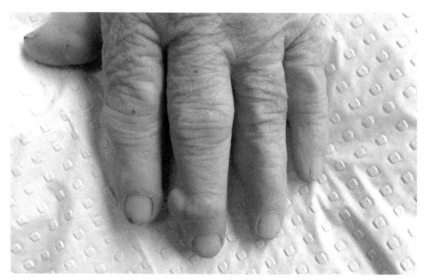

*Rheumatoid nodules on fingers.*

## Lumpy Rheumatoid
Published April 18, 2014

It's been a while since I've seen these many lumps on a rheumatoid arthritis (RA) patient.

He's had not-so-well controlled RA for decades and just presented from St Elsewhere.

These lumps are rheumatoid nodules. They are firm and felt under the skin, usually close to joints, and often close to areas which get exposed to trauma for example the hands, knuckles, and elbows.

Often you can move the nodules but sometimes, the nodules are firmly connected to the tissues under the skin.

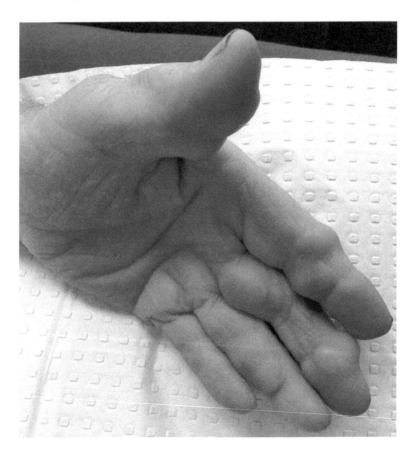

Rheumatoid nodules can also be found in areas distant from joints — the lungs, heart and other internal organs.

They can range in size, think a pea to a walnut. They can be painless but some people find them uncomfortable and irritating, particularly if they get bumped a lot.

Rheumatoid nodules are thought to be present in up to 20%-30% of RA patients, and are thought to be associated with more severe disease. Most patients with rheumatoid nodules have a positive rheumatoid factor (RF).

Smoking is thought to increase nodules. Methotrexate use has uncommonly been linked to increased development of rheumatoid nodules.

I don't get to see these very often nowadays, certainly not in 20-30% of my RA patients. Maybe it's because I get to see patients relatively early in their disease course or our treatments are more effective. I don't know.

I need to bring up the topic of fatigue as this, for some, is the most debilitating of symptoms. Many rheumatologists, including myself, do not have very effective ways of dealing with this. This post discusses it in more detail.

## What to do about overwhelming fatigue in rheumatology?
Published November 18, 2016

*ACR Scientific Meeting, Washington DC, November 2016:*

It's fair to say that most of us rheumatologists find it very hard to deal with the fatigue our patients have to deal with. As a result, many of us tend not to ask about it or we gloss over it.

And yet, for our patients, it's often a very major issue.

To try and learn more, I attended a session presented by Sarah Hewlett, Professor of Rheumatology Nursing, from the University of the West of England.

She gave us a snapshot of a large body of work and I'll try to distill what notes I managed to take in my jeglagged state.

With rheumatoid arthritis patients, 65% actually prioritised fatigue as most important, a higher number than those who prioritised pain.

Yet, I think most of us rheumatologists tend to focus on pain when we ask our questions.

Fatigue is just so common among all manner of patients, but for those with rheumatoid and other autoimmune conditions, it's appears "different to normal tiredness".

Descriptions include the "body feels heavy", "I struggle to get going", "I just don't have the strength".

It's a physical issue with a cognitive component.

Patients describe feeling as though they're moving in "Mud or Porridge". "Brain fog" is very common.

Fatigue often leads to people withdrawing from daily, social activities. How much the fatigue will affect them on any given day may be unpredictable. Withdrawal then leads to altered roles and relationships.

In some, the fatigue is overwhelming, and this leads to an emotional response.

In most, fatigue is frustrating as "no-one understands". It's "invisible".

In most cases, we're just not sure what causes the fatigue. It's likely to be down to a range of factors. Perhaps the disease being active, perhaps some combination of medication side effects. It might even result from the adjustment to having a chronic, incurable disease, or from becoming deconditioned as a result of changed activity due to having such a disease.

We need to support self-management of fatigue, so Professor Hewlett described an 8 stage process she uses:

- Validate the patient's experience. "Tell me what this fatigue is like for you...." "...other patients have told me...."

- Review & identify causes: deconditioning, sleep, doing too much, stress & anxiety, pain & disease activity, hunger, low mood.

- Use daily activity diaries & review regularly:

- Colouring a daily activity chart hour by hour really gives one an idea of how much we all do.

- It's not the nature of the task they are colour coding, it's colour coding how they feel while doing the task.

- Colours can be given for high energy activity vs low energy activity vs chill out/refresh time vs sleep vs crash.

- This visual aid will help patients process what they might need to do, to pace their lives.

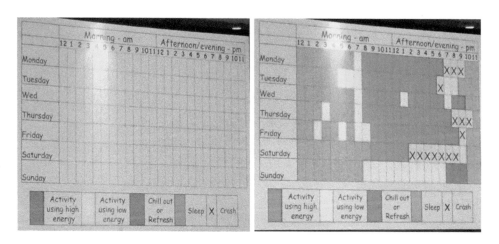

- Address boom & bust behaviour, the phenomenon of doing as much as possible on a "good" day in anticipation of likely having a "bad" day soon, with this overzealous activity leading to a "crash". A self-fulfilling cycle.

- Goal setting:

  Introduce the need to prioritize components of the wheel of life: eg learning, health, spiritual life, finance, family, etc.

  Then set goals to achieve priorities with the goals being specific, measurable, achievable, realistic, time-limited (SMART).

- Address deconditioning

- Tackle stress

- Improve sleep

I learned stuff that I hope will improve my practice.

Do you think the above suggestions might be useful?

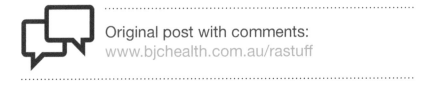

Original post with comments:
www.bjchealth.com.au/rastuff

# Chapter 3

There isn't a single test to diagnose rheumatoid arthritis. The diagnosis is made from a combination of clinical symptoms and findings, supported by various investigations.

Sometimes the diagnosis is clear cut. Sometimes, the way it presents is less typical with the diagnosis unclear and it might take some time to become more obvious.

Investigations may include blood tests such as rheumatoid factor (RF), anti-cyclic citrullinated peptide antibodies (anti-CCP) and elevated inflammatory markers. However, up to 30% of patients have completely normal blood tests.

RF testing is actually testing for a group of non-specific antibodies. While they can be found in up to 70% of patients diagnosed with RA, they can also occur in healthy people who will never get rheumatoid arthritis. RF can be elevated in many diseases such as hepatitis, chronic infection or other inflammatory diseases.

The level of RF can fluctuate during the course of disease but the actual level does not correlate with how active the disease may be. The RF does not typically normalise with treatment. This means that if you have RA, it is not necessary to monitor the RF regularly.

Anti-CCP antibodies, also known as ACPA are much more specific for RA. By that, I mean that a positive anti-CCP result will typically be highly suggestive that RA is the diagnosis. A negative anti-CCP result however does not rule out the disease as these antibodies are not found in all patients.

A positive anti-CCP result tends to be suggestive of a potentially more serious and destructive disease (if not controlled by appropriate treatment).

**Seropositive RA refers to the presence of RF and/or anti-CCP antibodies in a person diagnosed with RA.**

**Seronegative RA refers to the situation where both antibodies are not elevated.**

Inflammatory markers such as the erythrocyte sedimentation ratio (ESR) and C-reactive protein (CRP) are often elevated during active disease and can be good markers to monitor treatment response.

The higher the level, the more active the disease is. However, both are also elevated during acute infection and care must be taken to interpret an elevated reading.

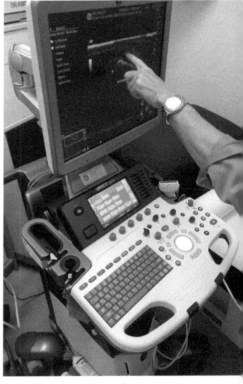

*Our ultrasound machine*

**To complicate things, the blood tests can be normal in some people with RA and the clinical features can be subtle.**

Your rheumatologist may then consider further investigations to look for active joint inflammation, such as magnetic resonance imaging (MRI) or a Power Doppler Ultrasound study to confirm the presence of active inflammation or erosion.

Erosions are caused by the aggressive tissue swelling or synovitis we've already mentioned. Erosions refer to the breaking down of bone around the joints that we can see on imaging studies. It's what we rheumatologists are trying to prevent with therapy.

X-rays of the joints may also be used, as they are cheaper and/or more accessible than MRI or power doppler ultrasound. X-rays however are normal in early disease, and are less sensitive in detecting early damage. X-rays are unable to show active inflammation.

**Normal X-rays do not exclude the diagnosis of rheumatoid arthritis.**

Rheumatologists often use a validated classification criteria to help with the diagnosis. This 2010 ACR/EULAR classification criteria provides a score for a number of clinical features and investigation results. A score of 6 or more leads to a definite classification of RA.

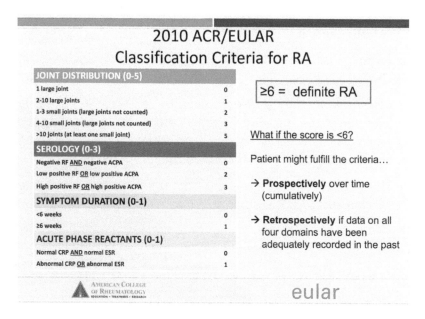

*Accessed 6th July 2016* - http://www.eular.org/myUploadData/files/ RA%20Class%20Slides%20ACR_Web.pdf

There is a worldwide move for rheumatologists to have access to ultrasound machines in their clinics. The improvements in technology with smaller sizes and lower costs have allowed this.

In Australia, around 20% of practicing rheumatologists are trained in ultrasound use. The rheumatologists at our clinic, BJC Health, routinely use this technology for RA so I've included a post on this:

## Will a pretty picture change your mind about your rheumatoid?
Published October 6, 2013

Sometimes, patients need convincing.

A rheumatologist's nimble fingers, good looks, and confident persona may not be sufficient.

Do I really have rheumatoid arthritis? Why do I need medication? I'm not that bad.

I like my ultrasound machine in these circumstances. I can show this patient what's happening at the joint level.

Seeing your body part on screen in real time is powerful. Watching the moving images while the probe moves against skin is justification. It's even more convincing when the "red flames" of inflammation flicker into view.

Here's a series of screenshots from my ultrasound machine of a patient with Rheumatoid Arthritis.

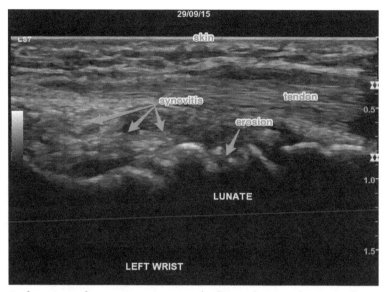

*Left wrist showing synovitis (inflamed tissue) as well as erosive change at the lunate bone.*

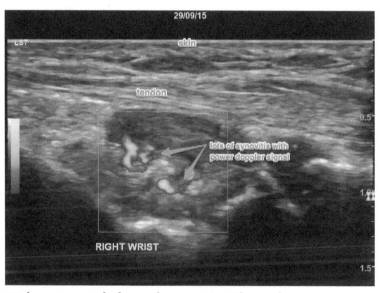

*Right wrist with lots of synovitis. The red represents an increase in power doppler signal representing abnormal blood vessels & active inflammation. This is usually associated with more aggressive disease.*

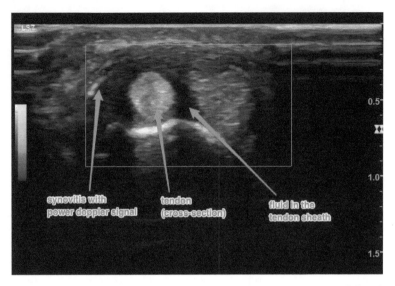

*This shows a tendon in cross section. There is increased fluid around the tendon as well as swollen tissue and increase in power doppler signal. This is consistent with tenosynovitis.*

Do you think this type of additional information is useful?

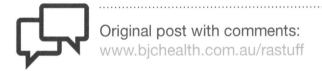

Original post with comments:
www.bjchealth.com.au/rastuff

# Chapter 4

## Treatment: How do we beat this disease?

If you have been given the diagnosis of rheumatoid arthritis, do not panic!

Over the last couple of decades, we have gained a lot of understanding about this disease, and what it takes to control the disease. There are now very effective medications.

The goal of treatment is to suppress the disease to prevent joint damage.

It is extremely important that RA is diagnosed early before the joints are damaged permanently.

Clinical evidence suggests early aggressive treatment results in a higher chance of achieving remission.

Your rheumatologist may use the term, the "**window of opportunity**", to describe this early period where there is the greatest opportunity to achieve the best results.

This window of opportunity is usually thought of as the first 6-12 months of the disease.

## The Window of Opportunity to EDUCATE about rheumatoid

Published December 8, 2013

I met her at the start of 2012. A young lady with a new husband.

She presented with a very swollen knee. The diagnosis was rheumatoid arthritis and it was an easy one to make, given she had very raised autoimmune serology (RF and anti-CCP) and her mother also had the disease.

They were trying for a baby so treatment options were limited. And it was just the one joint involved, so treatment was localised to aspiration and cortisone injection.

I think I got to see her three times. Then she disappeared. She cancelled a follow-up appointment, said she'd reschedule, and didn't.

In a busy rheumatology clinic, it's hard to have a good follow-up system for patients who don't want to return. And, I forgot about her.

She's now back. And the rheumatoid is rampant.

Over 21 months since review and she now has over 20 joints involved, both big and small. Her fingers are all deviated at the MCP joints (knuckles), her wrist movements are restricted and her thumbs are shaped like a Z.

The window of opportunity to switch off her rheumatoid is well and truly over. We missed it.

I had a window period to educate her on how serious her disease could potentially become. I missed that.

I figure all rheumatologists would spent a lot of time up front trying to explain this beast called rheumatoid arthritis. I thought I was relatively effective at this but this sort of occurrence brings me back to earth.

Why didn't she return?

Well, she was still trying to fall pregnant. And she thought that as long as she was trying, she couldn't be treated. I suspect she has had difficulty coping with having a chronic disease and just plodded along, accepting her symptoms. Even now in the face of very active, deforming rheumatoid, she tells me she is coping and has little pain.

I feel disappointed and sad at what's happened.

Especially as it was likely to have been preventable.

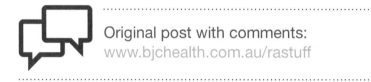

Original post with comments:
www.bjchealth.com.au/rastuff

## Medications

There are two main groups of medications commonly used to treat RA:

1.  **Anti-inflammatory medication** such as non-steroidal anti-inflammatory drugs (NSAIDs), cyclooxygenase-2 (Cox-2) inhibitors and corticosteroids (both oral and injected):

    a.  These are effective in controlling the symptoms but they are likely not effective in preventing joint destruction.

    b.  They work rapidly and most patients experience improvement within a few days.

    c.  They are typically gradually tapered once the symptoms improve because long term use of NSAIDs, Cox-2 inhibitors and especially, corticosteroids such as Prednisone may cause increasing side effects.

d. Examples of NSAIDs are Diclofenac (brand names include Voltaren and Fenac), Naproxen (brand names include Naprosyn and Anaprox), Ibuprofen (brand names include Advil and Nurofen), and many others.

e. The most commonly used Cox-2 inhibitor is Celexocib (brand name, Celebrex).

2. **Disease modifying anti-rheumatic drugs (DMARDs)** are medications, which work to help regulate the disordered immune system:

   a. **Conventional synthetic DMARDs** include Methotrexate, Sulphasalazine, Hydroxychloroquine, Leflunomide, Azathioprine, Gold, and Cyclosporin. They have different side effect profiles and all must be monitored closely.

   b. Only 30-50% of patients have adequate disease control with one agent and the majority of patients require combination treatment utilising a number of DMARDs.

   c. Over the last two decades, we have had a number of sophisticated medications genetically engineered to work on specific targets in the immune system. These are called **biologic DMARDs (bDMARDs)**.

   d. Even more recently, powerful oral medications have been developed to work within the immune cells, to disrupt the cell-signalling processes which lead to the inflammatory and immune responses seen in RA. These are called **targeted synthetic DMARDs**.

Very few rheumatologists would be using Azathioprine, Gold or Cyclosporin for RA these days given the poorer risk and benefit balance of these medications and the fact that there are better alternatives.

Widely used conventional synthetic DMARDs in RA would be Methotrexate (brand names, Methotrexate or Methoblastin), Sulphasalazine (brand name, Salazopyrin EN), Leflunomide (brand name, Arava) and Hydroxychloroquine (brand name, Plaquenil).

**By far, the most commonly used DMARD is Methotrexate. It is the medication most rheumatologists would start with in most patients at the time of RA diagnosis.**

If you are reading this book, chances are you will already have had to contemplate this medication.

Methotrexate does however suffer from stigma. I think this stems from the fact it has been used as chemotherapy to treat a variety of cancers as well as the very cautious approach that doctors appropriately took early in the use of Methotrexate.

So, I'm going to share a series of blog posts to help demystify this crucial medication.

## In my hands, Methotrexate is NOT chemotherapy
Published October 10, 2012

Methotrexate is a very useful medication. Rheumatologists would all agree. We use it for rheumatoid arthritis and many other types of autoimmune conditions.

I'm comfortable with it and have hundreds of patients on this medication.

Everyday, I spend a proportion of my time looking at Methotrexate-monitoring blood tests for patients using this medication. Every week, I would write a number of prescriptions.

It's also true that I would regularly spend a lot of time allaying patient fears about this drug.

Why?

Bad press. And misinformation. Lots of it.

Methotrexate has been used as chemotherapy at much, much higher doses and in different formulations than those used in arthritis. This leaves it with a stain. A little knowledge is a dangerous thing and many friends, family members, well-wishing members of the community, and even, some health professionals are guilty of scaremongering.

When rheumatologists use Methotrexate in the context of arthritis, it is NOT chemotherapy. It's an arthritis drug.

In fact, the doses we use, which are much lower, with the medication used once weekly only, and orally in the majority, are typically well-tolerated.

I am not saying that Methotrexate should not be used with caution or that its side-effect free.

Every medication has POTENTIAL side effects. As doctors, we would prescribe a medication if the potential benefits of the medication outweigh the potential risks of that medication.

We also monitor the patient's clinical state as well as blood tests closely to ensure safety. Side effects if they develop can be dealt with quickly and if necessary, the dose is reduced or the medication ceased. All it takes is good communication between patient and rheumatologist.

I write this post because of the many patients who are dissuaded from taking Methotrexate due to some scary thing they've read or been told about.

Typically, if your rheumatologist has suggested Methotrexate, there's a good reason. In the case of rheumatoid arthritis, it's because rheumatoid arthritis is a serious disease with many bad consequences when it's not treated adequately. Methotrexate is the initial, go-to drug in most cases.

What stories about Methotrexate have you heard?

## Ridiculous Things said about Methotrexate

Published March 17, 2013

I had to take a call from a patient I had just commenced on Methotrexate (at a low dose of 10 mg once a week).

She was worried by what a well-meaning friend and a well-intentioned pharmacist told her.

She was told that she needed to avoid contact with pregnant women! You can imagine how this made her feel. What a horrible drug Dr Lim was putting her on.

In addition, she could no longer take her Celebrex, the anti-inflammatory medication she was using to get some relief. How was she going to cope? Especially as Dr Lim had told her that Methotrexate would take upwards of 4 weeks to have effect. Cruel.

She wasn't actually told to stop the drug but she was warned strongly of potential problems with using the Celebrex while on Methotrexate. By the way, this combination is a common one and the combination of Methotrexate with pain relief medications and with anti-inflammatory medications is used widely and is generally safe.

Methotrexate, at the doses used in rheumatology is NOT chemotherapy but it suffers a stigma.

I'm glad she called so that I could discuss and correct the "information" she'd been given. I'm glad she didn't just decide never to take Methotrexate.

Over the years, my patients have reported a number of disturbing things told to them about Methotrexate:

1. You need to use a different toilet from other members of your family.

2. You need to use gloves to handle the tablets . Worse still, one patient who was hospitalised told me that the nurse

gowned up and wore gloves to hand her the Methotrexate tablet! With another, the staff at the local pharmacy refused to load her Methotrexate into the pill box citing occupational health & safety issues.

3. You have to avoid crowded, public places to avoid catching an infective disease

4. Fear mongering: It will kill you! It's poison! etc etc

Of course, Methotrexate has possible side effects. It's a serious drug and is treated as such. Doctors typically prescribe it when the potential benefits outweigh the risks (as should be the case with all medications).

But, misinformation abounds.

What ridiculous things have you been told about Methotrexate?

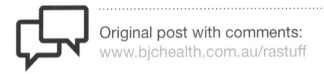

Original post with comments:
www.bjchealth.com.au/rastuff

## How I prescribe Methotrexate step-by-step
Published July 22, 2013

I started a couple of patients on Methotrexate today and did so the previous workday. I'm very likely to have to explain the drug tomorrow.

It's our go-to drug in rheumatology due to it's favourable benefit-risk ratio.

I thought it worth giving you some insight into how I go about explaining and prescribing this drug.

Please note that this is my general spiel and that there are many variations by rheumatologists all over the world. I also vary it depending on the actual patient and their other medical issues/ medications.

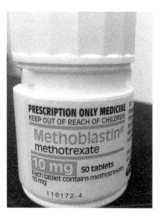

This is the gist of what I say:

1.  You may hear/read that Methotrexate is Chemotherapy and this might scare you. It's not chemotherapy & can be used safely. I explain why.

2.  We need to discuss the amount of alcohol you drink. I typically don't expect patients to become teetotallers, but I'm not comfortable with more than 1-2 standard drinks 2-3 nights a week (I do appreciate that what a patient admits to drinking & the reality may be different).

3.  I use 10 mg tablets. Commence Methotrexate at 10 mg ONCE A WEEK only at dinner time. If tolerated without any side effects (and patients are asked to contact me if there are any ill effects), the dose will then be increased to 20 mg ONCE A WEEK only.

4.  The day after the Methotrexate dose, you'll take 5 mg of folic acid (ie once weekly to start). This is used to reduce side effects.

5.  In about 3.5 weeks, after 4 doses (sooner if I am concerned about other medical issues/medications), the 1st monitoring blood tests will be performed. I usually see the patient 1 month after the commencement of Methotrexate.

Patients contemplating/commencing Methotrexate are emailed links to web-based resources to explain the medication. Where possible, my patients also now come in for further education with our rheumatology care coordinator, Flora (we think/feel/believe that the more education a patient has upfront, the better compliance & hopefully, understanding).

Again, note that my spiel and regime for commencing may be different from other rheumatologists. Some differences may be:

1. Different formulation of Methotrexate. Some rheumatologists prefer or only have access to a 2.5 mg tablet (rather than the 10 mg tablet).

2. Different preference for starting dose. Some may start Methotrexate at a lower dose, eg 7.5 mg once a week (ie 3 x 2.5 mg tablets).

3. Different speeds for increasing the dose.

4. Different formulations and regimes for folic acid use, ranging from 0.5 mg daily to 5 mg once weekly to 5 mg daily. I am not aware of any studies suggesting an optimum dose but it's accepted that using some folic acid reduces side effects.

5. Regimes are often tweaked depending on a patient's specific situation i.e individualised therapy.

I continue to write about Methotrexate to demystify and debunk myths. I hope this helps in some way. Please do feel free to share your thoughts.

## 6 Reasons why I stop Methotrexate
Published August 20, 2013

If you've been a reader of this blog, you'll know that Methotrexate is a go-to drug for rheumatologists.

It's considered safe, in the hands of rheumatologists and with monitoring.

It's considered the cornerstone of effective treatment for rheumatoid arthritis, it's a standard medication for psoriatic arthritis, and we often use it for its "steroid-sparing" effect (to reduce the need for steroid).

But, not everyone can tolerate it.

It's important patients know this. There are alternatives and I don't expect my patients to accept side effects which are significant to them, or to me.

When I think about it, the reasons/situations I would stop Methotrexate include:

1.  Side effects that worry a patient. Such as nausea or hair loss.

2.  Serious side effects that worry me. For eg, a rare reaction such as lung irritation/inflammation.

3.  Abnormal blood tests. Usually worsening liver function tests over time.

4.  Infections. I would normally withhold Methotrexate if there is a significant infection eg a pneumonia, and I would stop the drug permanently if recurrent infections occur.

5.  Patient Concern. Some worry so much about the drug, and even though I may not agree with the degree of worry, I don't think it's worth persisting with a medication if a patient is experiencing mental anguish.

6.  Inefficacy. There's no point persisting with a therapy that does not seem to be working (except that Methotrexate may be useful in combination with other drugs).

Have you had to stop Methotrexate for any other reason?

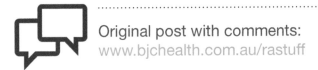

Original post with comments:
www.bjchealth.com.au/rastuff

## How long will I have to take this Methotrexate?
Published June 23, 2013

I was asked this question on Friday, I was asked earlier in the week, I've been asked before and I'm sure I'll be asked again.

Methotrexate, as the go-to drug for rheumatologists is something we discuss all the time with patients. It continues to amaze me how much misinformation there is about this medication.

The answer is pretty straightforward, and likely similar to the answer for any drug used long-term to treat a chronic disease.

My standard spiel:

**For as long as it works really well in controlling the disease**
and
**it doesn't cause you to have any side effects that worry you (or me)**
and
**there are no abnormalities in any of the monitoring tests we will do.**

Basically, the potential benefits must outweigh the potential risks.

If and when that situation changes, we reconsider. Often, we stop the medication and try another option if still required.

What have you been told about a long-term medication when you ask such a question?

Patients may have RA which is not controlled sufficiently well on Methotrexate as a sole DMARD. In this scenario, it is common for Methotrexate to be used in combination with other DMARDs.

We will discuss the use of combinations of different medications further in the chapter entitled *Strategy & Biologics*.

# Chapter 5

## The Possibility of Remission

While it's not nice to hear about the negative aspects of having RA, you need to have an appreciation of what happens to those with more aggressive disease. History has taught us certain lessons and this has led to an increasingly proactive and aggressive approach to treat RA.

**Put simply, for there to be a possibility of remission, we need to turn off the inflammation as quickly as possible and to calm down an immune system that is attacking its own host body.**

In the following blog posts, I try to highlight the changing attitudes and the better outcomes that we are now clearly achieving.

### Why I treat RA aggressively?
Published June 13, 2011

Up to 20% of patients with Rheumatoid Arthritis (RA) have a relatively good prognosis, with occasional flares and low level disease.

However, the majority with RA have progressive disease. This leads to joint destruction.

Destruction then deformity lead to suffering.

The reasons I and most other rheumatologists would treat rheumatoid arthritis aggressively (in the appropriate patient) is because rheumatoid arthritis is a 'bad' disease:

1. Patients with RA have a 1 in 3 chance of becoming disabled

2. Disability starts early:

    a. Within 1 year, 7.5% of patients will be unable to work at full capacity

    b. Within 10 years, 27% of RA patients were work disabled.

3. Mortality (death) is increased 2-fold for RA patients.

4. Mortality associated with RA is similar to that of diabetes. This risk of premature death is linked to the severity of RA.

5. RA is associated with a shortening of life expectancy by 7-10 years.

6. Patients with RA have an increased risk of developing other serious conditions, including:

    a. Infections, particularly lung, skin & joint infections;

    b. Lymphomas;

    c. Cardiovascular disease.

Given patients with uncontrolled disease do worse, our treatment strategies for rheumatoid arthritis now recognise that early therapy is critical.

Even a delay of as little as a few months in the introduction of disease-modifying anti-rheumatic drugs (DMARDs) following diagnosis can result in substantially more joint damage compared with early treatment.

Current thinking would suggest a strategy of intensive treatment. This includes:

1. Education for patients, about the disease & the therapies involved;

2. Early institution of DMARD therapy, with the 1st line choice usually Methotrexate;

3. The escalation of DMARD therapy from a single agent to triple therapy or alternative agents, including biologic DMARDs where required;

4. More frequent assessment of patients, utilising objective disease measures where possible;

5. Tight control of disease is the goal;

6. Multidisciplinary care utilising a rheumatology educator/nurse, physiotherapists, hand therapists, etc when required. These are elements of our Connected Care approach.

Rheumatologists are the specialty group with expertise in treating rheumatoid arthritis.

Early referral to a rheumatologist for early diagnosis, and appropriate DMARD therapy, are the cornerstones of successful treatment of RA.

Is this how your rheumatoid arthritis is being treated?

## An Easy Case of Rheumatoid
Published November 12, 2013

My rheumatology colleague, Andrew Jordan just presented a rheumatoid arthritis case at our GP meeting.

A 60-something year-old lady presenting with swelling and pain involving the small joints of her hands. Early morning stiffness and some carpal tunnel symptoms. A pretty classic story.

The diagnosis was made even easier by the presence of an elevated rheumatoid factor in her blood tests, and raised inflammatory markers.

The GP was astute and referred her early. She presented to a rheumatologist within 2 months of the onset of her symptoms.

Methotrexate was commenced with a small dose of Prednisone to help calm her symptoms. Within a few weeks, Prednisone had been weaned and ceased. She continued only on Methotrexate and was doing well.

One and a half years since her presentation, she remains in remission, both from her point of view and from the point of view of DAS-28 remission. She is symptom-free with absence of synovitis, the swelling rheumatologists look for when they examine joints.

All this on Methotrexate alone. 2 small tablets (10 mg each) once a week only.

Easy.

This is a near-perfect example of the window-of-opportunity.

Rob Russo (another rheumatologist) then made a telling comment. A decade or two ago, it would be strange to talk about an "easy" case of rheumatoid.

And of course, many cases don't pan out like this. Some patients have terribly aggressive disease. Sometimes, there are all sorts of logistical issues preventing early rheumatology review and early treatment.

There's a lot of debate currently about the very expensive treatments we use for rheumatoid.

There are massive cost savings to be had if we can treat patients early.

Within this window-of-opportunity, Methotrexate, a very cheap medication, works well for those who tolerate it.

Within this window-of-opportunity, this difficult disease becomes somewhat easier.

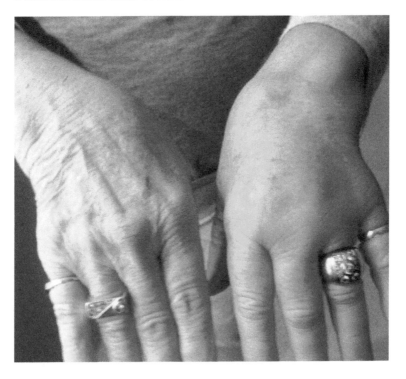

## The Goal Posts for Rheumatoid have moved
Published January 10, 2013

Once a month, the local rheumatologists meet at our tertiary level, teaching hospital to discuss challenging cases. We invite the patients being discussed to attend. Usually, there's a question being asked, a problem to resolve or sometimes, it's just cathartic for the patient and treating rheumatologist to efficiently get a range of opinions.

It was my turn.

My patient presented when she was 30 with an abrupt onset of rheumatoid arthritis. More than 20 joints swollen and inflamed, high inflammatory markers, very high autoantibody levels (both RF and anti-CCP). She was struggling to cope with daily life.

Bad disease. By any definition.

Over 6 years, I treated her with a variety of medications: Methotrexate, Prednisone, intra-articular steroid, Arava. Within 10 months of her symptoms, she was on biologic DMARD therapy. She has trialled Humira, Actemra, Orencia, Enbrel, and is now on Mabthera.

She has responded and is of course better than when she presented. But she has never entered sustained remission.

It's hard to tell that she has rheumatoid when you meet her.

She doesn't have the classical hand deformity. Her MRI of the hands do not show any active disease or erosive change affecting the fingers.

When you feel the swelling at both her wrists, see her wince a little, and note that she has lost a lot of movement at these joints, you then understand that the disease has caused damage and it's still affecting everything she does.

I presented her to see if the others could think of anything else to improve the situation.

Among the 6 rheumatologists present, there was over 100 years of clinical experience.

The consensus was that we had done well. A patient presenting the way she did, would in a previous era, be riddled with arthritis and deformity by now. She would very likely not still be working full time.

That might be true but I still feel that we should have done better. Rheumatologists are continuing to strive for better and better outcomes for our patients with rheumatoid arthritis.

The goal posts have moved, and during my career, I expect them to move much further.

There are various ways to define remission.

Rheumatologists have derived various measurements to help define this. If any of you have looked into clinical trial articles, or medical news sites, the most commonly referred to would be DAS-28 remission. Others include CDAI-remission, SDAI-remission and Boolean remission. These include components of the joint examination, the blood test results and assessments of how patients with RA feel to come up with some composite score. Having a scoring system then provides us with target numbers to aim for.

I think most patients think of remission very differently. For someone with RA, remission should probably be a state of not having the disease affect them in any way. They feel well, without joint pain or stiffness, and without other related symptoms. They don't have any side effects and for all intents and purposes, they can just get on with their lives normally.

We do have opportunity to provide such a remission for some, albeit with the help of various medications.

# Chapter 6

## Strategy & Biologics

*Please note that this chapter delves into greater depth with the newer therapies we have. If you are just commencing your RA education, you might want to skim or skip this chapter, leaving the detail for a later date.*

In the last chapter, I wanted to explain that we, rheumatologists and patients, now have different goals with RA.

We want to achieve remission where possible.

This might not be possible in people who present after years of less well-controlled disease, as it's already highly likely that the abnormal immune responses have already become deep-seated and established.

In this case, we try to achieve the lowest level of disease activity as possible. We also should be striving to achieve the best quality of lives for people we are trying to help.

How do we actually attain this?

I would love to say that treatment of RA is very precise, that we can measure stuff in the blood or stool or get some genetic analysis of skin or hair, and then design the best treatment regime based on the findings, specific to the individual.

Treatment of RA is not like this. Not yet.

At the moment, there are some clear cookbook recipes.

For example, the majority of us rheumatologists will commence Methotrexate when the diagnosis is made, if there are not good reasons not to.

If Methotrexate does not seem to be working to control the disease sufficiently well, other DMARDs are used in combination with Methotrexate.

If the disease is very severe at the time of diagnosis and there are markers suggesting that it will be aggressive, many rheumatologists may even commence 2 or 3 DMARDs straight away.

In Australia, the most common conventional DMARDs used in all variety of combinations include Methotrexate, Hydroxychloroquine (Plaquenil), Sulphasalazine (Salazopyrin EN) and Leflunomide (Arava).

We monitor our patients regularly and we adjust therapy as needed to control the disease, or to get rid of unwanted side effects, and to achieve our shared goals.

The following posts should give you some sense of these strategies.

## With RA, WHEN is more important than WHAT
Published December 8, 2012

I'm currently in Leeds, UK, visiting Chapel Allerton Hospital. This hospital is home to the Section of Musculoskeletal Disease, a world-renowned clinical academic rheumatology group.

20 rheumatologists from around the world were invited to a course run by the rheumatologists at this leading centre, chaired by Professor Paul Emery. We discussed aspects of rheumatoid arthritis and were encouraged to pick the brains of the Leeds team.

The 1st discussion made enough of an impression to trigger this post.

With rheumatoid arthritis, WHEN you treat is probably more important than WHAT you use to treat?

What do I mean by this statement?

Well, there is clearcut evidence that early diagnosis and therefore early, appropriate treatment of rheumatoid arthritis makes a huge difference to the quality of a patient's life, both in the short and long term.

It is therefore the onus of a rheumatology service to invest in a system for early referral.

Even this renowned rheumatology unit at Leeds needed to start out by trying to get GPs to refer patients early. Many letters to the surrounding 1000s of GPs have been sent, trying to educate and hammer home the message. Lots of talks have been presented and key patient advocacy groups mobilised.

Early arthritis should be treated as an "emergency". The quicker the referral, the quicker treatment is instituted once a diagnosis of rheumatoid arthritis is made, the better the outcomes for the patient, and the health service.

Time from symptom onset to control of disease activity needs to be improved.

We rheumatologists spent so much time arguing the various pros and cons of the different medications we have available to use. We ponder so much about what combinations are best, and we argue over different treatment algorithms to improve the effectiveness of these medications.

But, we also really need to spend time working out how we get the patient who develops symptoms of inflammatory arthritis to see their primary doctor earlier. We then need to work out how we empower this general practitioner to refer to his/her favourite rheumatology service ASAP. And, we need to ensure that the rheumatology service is set-up to be able to fast track review of these patients.

Rheumatologists will need to work harder on strategies to overcome various roadblocks affecting the above.

The WHEN needs to be as quick as possible.

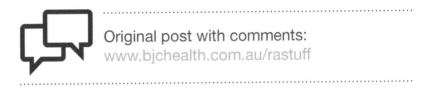

Original post with comments:
www.bjchealth.com.au/rastuff

# Biologic DMARDs

If combination therapy with the conventional oral DMARDs does not provide sufficient control of the disease, biologic DMARDs (bDMARDs) will need to be considered.

bDMARDs (ie Humira, Enbrel, Remicade, Simponi, Cimzia, Orencia, Actemra and Mabthera) are more powerful immuno-suppressants and are given as either subcutaneous injections or regular infusions through veins.

It has been more than a decade since people with RA in Australia have had access to biologic DMARD medications, with the costs heavily subsidised by our government.

This has been a massive advance for rheumatologists in achieving better outcomes and of course, it has been a boon to people with the disease who have not been doing well enough on the conventional DMARDs.

The problem is the high monetary costs of these agents.

While it's unsavoury for some to have to compromise on treatment due to cost, this is an increasing reality given the limited health dollar in all nations.

Strategies to use these high cost, highly effective medications in the most efficient and cost-effective manner are needed.

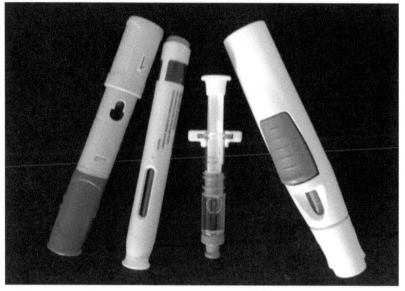

*Subcutaneous bDMARDs: Humira, Enbrel, Orencia, Simponi*

## With so many biologics for rheumatoid, how do you choose?
Published December 12, 2012

I'm over the jet lag. I think. The brain fog lifted sometime this AM.

The 2 days I spent in Leeds discussing rheumatoid arthritis with 20 rheumatologists from around the world seems like a blur.

One key discussion point needs review and I write down my thoughts today, to help you understand but also to force me to document this before I forget!

In Australia, we are lucky enough to have access to 8

biologic DMARDs once a patient with rheumatoid arthritis is deemed to have severe enough disease and has jumped through a range of hoops to meet set criteria. Now, it would be really nice to be able to work out which medication would be most useful for that individual patient sitting in front of me.

People, patients, respond differently to different therapies. Clinical trial results tell you about how a group responds. Not specifically about the patient sitting in front of me. Of course, we use the scientific evidence that we have to try to make an educated guess. But, it's sometimes not so easy.

With this in mind, I asked the question.

## How do you choose what biologic to use?

This diverse group of rheumatologists were from the UK, Spain, Finland, Germany, Russia, Kuwait, Israel, Brazil, Mexico, Columbia, Poland and Australia. There were clinicians and researchers, young and old, those who worked in the public hospital system and those in private practice.

The following is a synthesis of what I took away from the discussion and my own evolving practice.

**Please do not take this as prescriptive.** There is insufficient clinical trial evidence to be certain and as new head-to-head trials are reported, my approach and choices will likely change.

1.  The 1st choice tends to be a TNF inhibitor, and the 2 used most commonly are Enbrel (Etanercept) and Humira (Adalimumab). This is not surprising given the TNF inhibitors were the 1st class of biologic agents available for rheumatoid arthritis. Enbrel and Humira were the 1st 2 subcutaneous agents, are generally effective and reasonably well tolerated with good patient registry data over the decade to monitor for safety. Rheumatologists, and doctors in general, tend to be creatures of habit, so it makes sense that they stick with what they know until

there is compelling evidence to make them change.

2. Remicade (Infliximab), which is a TNF inhibitor that is given intravenously, is used more in places/centres where there is easy access to infusion rooms.

3. If the patient does not respond at all to the TNF inhibitor (primary failure), most would change the class of biologic agent. By this, I mean that they would use a non-TNF inhibitor. The choices are Mabthera (Rituximab), Actemra (Tocilizumab), Orencia (Abatacept). Which of these will be used first up after TNF inhibitor failure is quite variable.

Please note that rheumatologists are skilled at taking into account many variables when making a choice.

For example, a rheumatoid patient can have other health issues which make the choice of medication, and in particular, biologic medication tricky.

4. If a patient has evidence of latent Tuberculosis (Tb) or is at very high risk of Tb exposure, we would typically treat with drugs to treat the Tb. These would be started prior to the commencement of biologic agent and then overlapped for some months. In the era prior to Tb prophylaxis becoming standard, there were less cases of Tb reported with Enbrel and so for some, that is the TNF inhibitor of choice when Tb is an issue. Some would prefer to use Mabthera as this medication does not seem to increase risk of Tb but most countries do not allow Mabthera to be used as 1st line treatment so access is difficult.

5. If there is a history of cancer, it is likely to be safe to use any of the agents if the cancer has been treated and not recurred for at least 5 years. Most however, were keen to use Mabthera (if it was able to be accessed) particularly if the cancer was non-Hodgkin's lymphoma as Mabthera is very effective for that condition.

6. If the patient has multiple sclerosis or a family history of such, most would generally avoid TNF inhibitor therapy (but it was noted that the evidence is still uncertain if there is a link between these agents and multiple sclerosis).

7. If there is evidence of skin or any other vasculitis, or an overlap syndrome (meaning that the patient seems to be having a combination of different autoimmune disease such as rheumatoid and lupus) or possibly in the setting of chronic leg ulcers, Mabthera would seem a good choice given it's B-cell directed mode of action.

8. When there is a high CRP, persistent anaemia, or elevated platelet counts, this may imply high levels of an inflammatory protein called IL-6. In that case, Actemra would probably be a good choice.

9. If the patient has Hepatitis B virus infection, we need to avoid Mabthera & there is probably no great option among the other agents in terms of being more safe. Typically, anti-viral treatment will be needed.

10. If the patient has Hepatitis C virus infection, the TNF inhibitors seem to be safe.

11. If a patient suffers from chronic infections such as bronchiectasis, most would try to avoid TNF inhibitors. A common choice would be Orencia given the feeling that this medication causes less infection.

12. When a patient has Interstitial Lung Disease, some would avoid TNF inhibitor therapy and try to access Mabthera instead.

13. If the patient already has a prosthetic joint, for eg, a knee replacement, some argued that this would be a relative contraindication for TNF inhibitor use as the infection risk is higher. Especially if, the patient also suffered with chronic leg ulceration.

14. Most agreed that Abatacept had a lower rate of infections. In some countries, this medication is not currently used much due to the current lack of availability of the subcutaneous formulation but this will change in the future.

15. Mabthera would be a good choice in patients who are seropositive (have positive RF and anti-CCP) and who have hypergammaglobulinemia (raised levels of a protein called IgG). This does not mean that these patients will not respond to the other agents. Just that these are the characteristics of patients who respond to Mabthera.

16. In patients who need treatment while attempting to fall pregnant, the TNF inhibitors are likely to be safe even if the pharmaceutical companies would be unlikely to actively encourage use in this subgroup of patients. Enbrel or Cimzia had been used among the group.

17. In very obese patients, subcutaneous biologic medications may not work as well.

It's complicated, isn't it?

I again highlight that these are certainly not guidelines. They represent a combination of evidence, some extrapolation of scientific principles, and the clinical experience of a range of rheumatologists.

I hope this gives you some insight as to the amount of thought that your rheumatologist puts into their decision making.

I'd love to hear the thoughts of my rheumatology colleagues reading this.

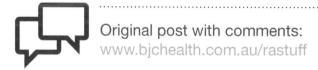

Original post with comments:
www.bjchealth.com.au/rastuff

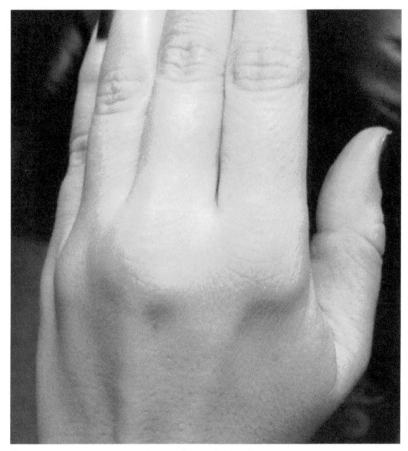

*Persistent synovitis at the 2nd & 3rd MCP joints*

In 2017, we have even more medication options. However, the choice of which biologic DMARD to start remains imprecise in most cases. This is something your rheumatologist will base on their experience, whether or not you have seropositive or sero-negative RA, your relevant other medical conditions, and what agents are accessible.

## If you need to fail 2 DMARDs before going onto a biologic, is that not missing the window of opportunity?

Published November 22, 2012

This post is written in response to a very perceptive question by a regular contributor to this blog, Naomi Creek.

I have previously written about the need for early, aggressive therapy in Rheumatoid Arthritis. This is because there appears to be a period early in the disease, when effective treatment will have its best chance for effect. In a real world setting, this leads to less longer term pain and suffering, less joint damage and therefore, less joint deformity.

This is referred to as the **Window of Opportunity.**

We don't know exactly how long this window period lasts but it's probably in the 1st 6-12 months of disease.

If that's the case, the question is how we take advantage of this period and how aggressive the treatment needs to be early on. Lots of current studies are being conducted to try and answer this.

A big issue is how to get patients starting to suffer these symptoms into a rheumatologist's rooms as soon as possible for the diagnosis to be made. An essential step before effective treatment is typically prescribed. This is a problem and will need a separate post, some other day.

Naomi asks:

"with the system here in Australia, patients cannot just go straight onto combined therapy [talking about biologic combo], so has their window of opportunity for remission gone?"

"If a patient has to fail two DMARDs before going onto a biologic — say at the 6 month mark, is that not missing the window of opportunity?"

My response:

The trials suggest that the **use of combination TNF inhibitor therapy and Methotrexate in early rheumatoid arthritis leads to better results than Methotrexate alone.** For example, the *OPTIMA study* or the *COMET study.*

The issue is cost. Most of our societies are not coping with the increasing costs of healthcare. And this needs to be contained.

So different strategies need to be considered and then tested in trials to help guide our real world decisions.

Take the OPTIMA study I mentioned above.

While it's true the use of Adalimumab/Methotrexate compared to Methotrexate led to better outcomes at the 6 month mark, the addition of Adalimumab to the group of patients treated with Methotrexate alone who did not have an adequate response at the 6 month mark then allowed this group to "catch up".

By that I mean, the longer term clinical and functional outcomes of both groups became comparable at 1 year and further.

This is good to see. It suggests that our current Australian system where we can only use a biologic at 6 months after the failure of 2 traditional DMARDs will still lead to good results.

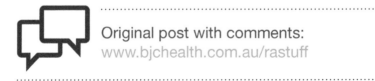

Original post with comments:
www.bjchealth.com.au/rastuff

## Is cheap, triple therapy as good as biologic therapy in RA?

Published June 27, 2013

A very important paper was recently published in the New England Journal of Medicine (http://www.nejm.org/doi/pdf/10.1056/NEJMoa1303006) and it has led to lots of interest.

The last decade in rheumatology has really been shaped by the biologic medication.

I think they have been a great advance and I argued previously how much they have changed the way we practice. Not just by using the new biologic medication but also in how we approach earlier diagnosis and better management strategies with our older drugs.

The major disadvantage of the biologic medications is COST. They cost heaps, upwards of $20,000 (Aus) per year and this is a major issue for all governments (and us taxpayers), rich or poor.

This study by O'Dell et al. compares a much cheaper option.

In patients with rheumatoid arthritis who are not well controlled enough on Methotrexate (MTX) alone,

- Half were given Salazopyrin EN (SSZ) and Hydroxychloroquine (HCQ) to be used in combination with MTX. This combo is known as Triple Therapy.

- Half were given Etanercept (Enbrel, ETA) to be used in combination with MTX

So, it was MTX/SSZ/HCQ vs MTX/ETA.

Over the first 24 weeks of the trial, both groups had comparable and significant improvement, based on the DAS28 (a disease activity score).

At 24 weeks, the patients with an inadequate response were switched to the other therapy, i.e. inadequate response to

MTX/SSZ/HCQ leads to a switch to MTX/ETA. About 27% of patients in each group needed to have this switch.

At 48 weeks, the responses were basically the same in both groups, in terms of disease activity improvements, functional improvement, quality of life scores, and major side effects.

This is good stuff!

My rough guess is a saving of A$15,000/yr for a similar result.

The major drawback of the triple therapy group is the pill load.

A MTX/SSZ/HCQ group will require MTX tablets weekly, up to 4 tablets of SSZ daily, and another 2 tablets of HCQ daily, in addition to the anti-inflammatory medication (NSAIDs + Prednisone). A MTX/ETA group would replace the daily SSZ/HCQ tablets with a once weekly subcutaneous injection.

This trial's a good one.

I feel it also shows the benefit of treating to target. If your pre-defined disease target is not reached, whether you're on biologic or triple therapy or some other combination, and there are no other medical reasons not so, the therapy should be switched to achieve a better outcome.

What do I currently do?

Well, I typically start with MTX to treat rheumatoid arthritis. If a patient does not seem to be responding well in the 1st few months, I usually add in HCQ or SSZ to work in combination with MTX. If by week 24 (or around this time), the patient has not improved sufficiently and has no other medical reasons not to, I usually move the patient on to a biologic agent in combination with MTX.

Over the years, I've used Triple Therapy less and less. But, I may be changing to use both HCQ and SSZ in combination with MTX more often. My bias has been that this combination, due to the pill load, is hard to "sell" to the patient and leads to more side effects. And if side effects occur, it's not easy to know which medication to blame!

But, the cost savings are compelling.

What do my rheumatology colleagues think? Will this study move us back to using more Triple Therapy?

## Triple Therapy vs Biologic/MTX: the debate rages
Published October 30, 2013

I've been following the American College of Rheumatology Meeting in San Diego on twitter.

There's been a fair bit of chatter regarding the relative merits of using Triple Therapy (Methotrexate/Sulphasalazine/Hydroxychloroquine) for Rheumatoid Arthritis compared to biologic therapy/Methotrexate therapy after the failure of Methotrexate as monotherapy.

I'd previously written about the thought-provoking O'Dell paper that has reignited this debate.

There's no denying that biologic therapy is really very expensive. All developed countries have budgets in deficit and the money printing will have to stop sometime. Health costs are soaring and we as rheumatologists are definitely adding to the bill.

This debate counts.

And yet, I must admit I haven't changed my practice yet.

I sit here trying to justify why this is the case to myself and the points I've come up with:

- Pill Load: With triple therapy, 2 or more tablets Methotrexate weekly, at least 1-7 tablets of folic acid weekly, 4 tablets of sulphasalazine daily, 2 tablets of hydroxychloroquine daily, add in some Prednisone early in the treatment cycle, possibly calcium and vitamin D supplementation, possibly fish oil. A patient will need at least 45-50 tablets a week.

- With the 1st point, compliance is likely to be poor. Sorry, but I find it hard to believe most of my patients will adhere to taking all these.

- Confusion. Mine. With different medication started together, it's harder to work out if and when a side effect occurs, which therapy to blame? To enable me to stop or modify it.

- The baseline characteristics of the patients in the trial reported seem different from mine. The patients had late disease, at a mean of 5 years post-diagnosis. They seem older than my usual group with an age mean around 57 years.

- The patients had been on Methotrexate as monotherapy for at least 12 weeks and were doing quite badly with a high mean DAS28 of 5.8, mean swollen joint score of 11 and mean tender joint score of 13. Our treat-to-target mantra would usually have meant some combination therapy would already have been started unless there were good reasons not to.

Now, I'm likely just justifying what I do.

I still try to treat aggressively and I still treat-to-target, seeing my Rheumatoid Arthritis patients regularly while aiming for remission or a state as close as possible to this. I use Methotrexate then add in Hydroxychloroquine and/or Salazopyrin EN early if our targets are not being met. I just don't tend to start the whole lot as described.

And yet, I do understand the financial imperative to use cheaper drugs if possible. After all, it's your tax dollars and it's my tax dollars.

If I had to pay and if you had to pay (rather than our funding bodies subsidising the treatments greatly), would we do something different?

The answer I think is (maybe) yes. We would use this triple therapy regime earlier. We would justify it better. Rheumatologists would cajole more.

And maybe, I won't need this introspective yet on-line discussion. My funding body, the government, may eventually take it out of my hands and mandate that we use triple therapy as described as part of the process to gain access to biologic medication.

These are my thoughts. What are yours?

## Biologic DMARDs have to get cheaper. Here's how.
Published November 2, 2013

I felt the need to write this follow up post.

The debate about Triple Therapy vs Methotrexate in rheumatoid arthritis exists due to the disparity of costs.

If both are similarly effective (it's debatable which types of patients this statement applies to), we really should be using the cheaper alternative much more.

If both were similarly priced, I don't think we'd be having this debate. I'm guessing most rheumatologists would choose the biologic/Methotrexate combo.

Wouldn't it be good then if the price differential reduces?

This will occur. I don't know how quickly or how much, but these are some ways:

## Competition

The rise of Biosimilars: patents for biologic DMARDs are expiring.

While these are difficult medications to copy due to their molecular size and the complexity of manufacture, there are medications being reverse engineered to look like and act like the original. Already, there are biosimilars for Inflix-imab, Etanercept and Rituximab. As these enter the market, I've heard estimates of 30%+ reduction in price.

## Use biologic DMARDs earlier in strategies that allow cessation of the biologic

We may one day be allowed to use the biologic/Methotrex-ate combination upfront with a plan once the rheumatoid arthritis is well controlled to then stop using the biologic and hopefully keep disease control using the cheaper med-ication.

The *OPTIMA trial* is an example of this. Rheumatoid patients with early disease (<1 year & naive to Methotrex-ate, and this may be a key point) were given Adalimumab/Methotrexate. After 26 weeks, roughly half of those who had good disease control had the Adalimumab stopped. At the end of the study after 78 weeks, the outcomes were similar between the group that stopped Adalimumab and the group that stayed on it.

## Reduction of the dose of biologic DMARDs

Once patients achieve good control of their disease, some rheumatologists and some patients may reduce either the amount of biologic medication being given. This leads to flare in some but in others, disease control remains good. There is limited trial data for this approach but it's a strategy likely to be explored.

Lower dose means less costs. Less frequent administration means less costs.

The *PRESERVE trial* is an example of this. The patient population was different to the OPTIMA trial, with later disease, and persistent, uncontrolled disease despite Methotrexate use.

Rheumatoid patients who received a low disease activity score on the Etanercept 50 mg weekly/Methotrexate combination were then randomised to one of three treatment groups: 50 mg Etanercept/Methotrexate, 25 mg Etanercept/Methotrexate, or placebo/Methotrexate.

The 2 groups using Etanercept, both the conventional & the reduced dose, maintained disease control better that the Methotrexate only group. The outcomes for the 2 different doses of Etanercept were about the same.

Thanks for all the comments regarding this topic on twitter and this forum. Please do continue to share your thoughts.

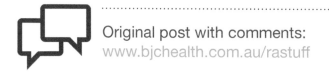

Original post with comments:
www.bjchealth.com.au/rastuff

Since that post, there has been accumulating evidence that we can use the most commonly used biologic DMARDs, TNF inhibitor medications, in early RA, control the underlying disease, and in those who respond well, take away the TNF inhibitors.

We also have some evidence that we can do the same with other biologic DMARDs used in early RA. Here's a blog post describing this strategy with Abatacept (Orencia).

## Can we use biologic DMARDs early then take them away?

Published December 8, 2014

Another one's here!

I recently wrote about a strategy trial using Etanercept very early in the treatment of rheumatoid arthritis followed by withdrawal of the drug.

This was a much anticipated trial providing insights which will help us use biologic DMARDs more strategically.

Well, we now have another similar strategy trial published.

This time using a biologic DMARD with a different mode of action, Abatacept. Abatacept is a fusion protein of cytotoxic T lymphocyte-associated antigen-4 and immunoglobulin G1. It selectively modulates a signal required for full T-cell activation (Etanercept by way of comparison, is a TNF inhibitor).

Here is the link to the journal article: the AVERT study at http://ard.bmj.com/content/annrheumdis/74/1/19.full.pdf (updated as study extended).

As a brief summary:

- The patients recruited had early disease (a mean symptom duration of 0.56 years). They had a high inflammatory burden (a mean swollen joint count of 11.1 and a mean CRP of 17.5 mg/L), as well as poor prognostic factors (all had positive anti-CCP with 95% also having a positive RF).

- Patients were randomised to Abatacept /Methotrexate (MTX) in combination vs Abatacept alone vs MTX alone.

- At month 12, the proportion of patients in these 3 groups achieving DAS28<2.6 (Disease activity score-defined remission) were 60.9% vs 42.5% vs 45.2%.

- These patients who achieved DAS28 remission then had their treatment stopped rapidly! Abatacept was withdrawn immediately and MTX (as well as any corticosteroids used) tapered over 1 month.

- At month 18, 6 months after withdrawal of therapy, 24.7% vs 28% vs 17% remained in DAS-defined remission.

These are encouraging results given the group of patients would be considered "difficult" as they had highly active disease at baseline with poor prognostic factors.

A durable remission following withdrawal of medication remains a holy grail in early rheumatoid arthritis. This trial seems another nice step towards this.

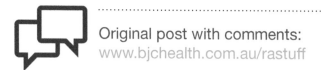

Original post with comments:
www.bjchealth.com.au/rastuff

As of April 2017, we have biosimilar Infliximab with the original medication being Remicade, as well as biosimilar Etanercept with the original medication being Enbrel, available to be prescribed in Australia.

## The TNF-inhibitor Biosimilar era is upon us. What is a biosimilar?
Published August 28, 2016

We've been lucky in Australia to have had access to biologic medication with a range of TNF-inhibitor medications since 2004 through a scheme where our government heavily subsidises the costs.

These medications are used to help those with inflammatory arthritis, such as rheumatoid arthritis, psoriatic arthritis and ankylosing spondylitis; skin disease (psoriasis);and/or inflammatory bowel disease.

You'll only qualify to access these medications if other conventional ("older") treatments have not adequately controlled the disease, and the major reason for this delay in access is the very high cost of these drugs. I'm not privy to the actual costs to the government but let's say it's in the order of $20,000 (Australian) each year per person.

Yup. Really expensive.

Enter the biosimilars.

As patents for medications expire, we typically have generic compounds become available. These are copies of the original drug made generally by other companies and brought to market at lower prices (in general). In general, the payer (eg government) saves money, and in theory, savings should pass on to end users and to tax payers.

Think of anti-cholesterol drugs or blood pressure medications. There are numerous generics as these drug molecules are relatively easy to copy and manufacture.

With TNF-inhibitor medications, it's not at all easy to create an identical copy. The molecules are very large and very complex. In addition, they are synthesised in a biological system i.e. reproduced within a cell, and this is a delicate and complicated procedure which can have variability at many different steps.

So, other companies have to reverse engineer a version of the original drug.

They have not been able to create an identical compound to date.

Instead, what is produced is a drug which is "biosimilar" to the original medication.

These medications then go through a series of tests and trials, to prove their safety and their "similarity" to the original medication in some of the clinical settings that the TNF-inhibitor medications are used in.

The results of these tests, for the biosimilar medications coming to market, have been good, good enough to convince authorities that they should be approved for use in a host of conditions that the original medications are being used in. There has been a degree of extrapolation.

Now, the big hope is that this will lead to cost savings.

It's also fair to say that there is a degree of misunderstanding and worry among patients using the original medications and among rheumatologists (and other prescribing doctors) facing a lot of new, "similar" but not identical drugs, over the next few years.

I previously mentioned a new class of powerful oral medications. These are called **targeted synthetic DMARDs.**

They are distinct from the biologic DMARD medications in how they work and with the fact that they are taken orally rather than as injections.

The 1st of these agents to be used in routine clinical practice is Tofacitinib (trade name: Xeljanz), a JAK inhibitor.

It has been developed to work within the immune cells, to inhibit proteins called kinases, to then disrupt the cell-signalling processes which lead to the inflammatory and immune responses seen in RA.

The following post is about Tofacitinib and another JAK inhibitor, Baricitinib.

## JAK inhibitors cometh
Published February 21, 2017

The New England Journal of Medicine (NEJM) paper published last week reminded me to write this post.

We've been lucky in Australia to have access to the JAK-inhibitor, Tofacitinib (trade name, Xeljanz). It's been a welcome addition to the medications we have available to treat rheumatoid arthritis.

Xeljanz has been used more widely than was expected and as I consider my own prescribing of the medication, there are clear reasons:

- It's a pill. Some people have a clear preference to take a medication orally rather than have an injection. This is somewhat opposed to my own bias if I had to use medications myself. I think I would personally like to avoid having to take daily medications and I would prefer an injection intermittently as long as the interval is long enough (biologic medication options used in rheumatology can be given 1 weekly, 2 weekly, 4 weekly & even 12 weekly in psoriatic arthritis).

- Many of the biologic medications used in rheumatoid arthritis seem to work better when used in combination with Methotrexate. Xeljanz can be used as monotherapy, that is, without Methotrexate. There is good trial evidence that it is still effective in this way. This makes it one of two choices (the other being Tocilizumab (trade name, Actemra)) for those who cannot tolerate or who don't want to take Methotrexate.

The NEJM paper presented the 52-week results for the BEAM trial where Baricitinib (a JAK 1, 2 inhibitor) was compared to Adalimumab (trade name, Humira).

1305 patients who had rheumatoid which was incompletely controlled on Methotrexate were randomised to receive either placebo, 4 mg daily of Baricitinib or Adalimumab 40 mg every fortnight.

Both Baricitinib and Adalimumab were clearly superior to placebo.

The exciting news was that Baricitinib performed better than Adalimumab in a number of outcome measures at various time points during the trial.

This is an important result and clearly shows how effective this oral medication is.

What we need now is longer term data to convince us that these medications are at least as safe or safer than the current biologic DMARDs in widespread use.

Many have bet that JAK inhibitor medications will play a big part in rheumatoid arthritis management.

Looks like they're going to be correct.

The link to the paper:

http://www.nejm.org/doi/full/10.1056/NEJMoa1608345

The future is exciting. And confusing.

It's fair to say that we are getting a whole new range of medications to use in RA and that over time, these should become more affordable especially when patents expire for the new oral targeted synthetic DMARDs (as they are much simpler and cheaper to make compared with biologic DMARDs).

We still however need to learn how to use what we have more sensibly.

The goal should be to use the right drug in the right person at the right time.

# Chapter 7

## Side Effects

It's really common for people to focus on side effects when the discussion turns to medication.

I am very open to a discussion about possible side effects with the emphasis on "possible".

Every medication is a potential "poison" so the decision to use medication should not be taken likely. Appreciation of risk of side effects is needed.

However, we also **need to get across an appreciation of the risk of not treating the disease properly.**

**Medications are used only when the potential benefits outweigh the potential risks.**

We then need to reconsider the decision if side effects actually occur. More minor side effects may be tolerated while more serious side effects will trigger a change in medication.

## Balancing Odds of Drug Working vs Chance of Side Effects

Published July 22, 2015

This is a conversation I thought I'd share as it seems to touch on very pertinent concerns.

As you know, I write a bit about Methotrexate as it seems to be quite a maligned drug. These posts are popular and this particular conversation took place on the comments section of *Why Methotrexate is My Current Go To Drug in Rheumatoid Arthritis.*

Rosiet is 8 months post-RA diagnosis and is at the point of contemplating Methotrexate.

**Rosiet:** "I am trying very hard to educate myself as I move through this disease. I am not sure yet if your words have comforted me to the degree of accepting the Methotrexate, but at least, it has given me more information."

While there is so much information on the internet, it can be so confusing for someone faced with a chronic illness.

They can read scary things about the disease. They can read scary things about medication.

They can read confusing and sometimes, contradictory info about a variety of treatments, potions, remedies and snake oils. They can also research medications, and get wildly different opinions.

I take this as a reminder that we rheumatologists need to keep improving information and resources for patients to access. Patient support associations also need to become more visible so that people looking online actually come across their services.

**Rosiet:** "And, what I am just figuring out is that none of these drugs have much of a 'success' rate nor longevity to them. I am understanding that odds for each drugs effectiveness are relatively low to a high chance of side effects and that after an amount of time they stop working … and, you have to spin the wheel again …"

I wrote back as I did not agree with that assessment but I can understand how someone trying to find information online can be led to that opinion.

Rheumatoid Arthritis is not one single disease that acts the same way in every patient.

There is variability of severity, there are different outcomes for different patients, there are differences in how well people respond to medications, and of course, side effects occur in some and not in many others.

So it's not that easy to determine the likely success rate of a particular medication in any one patient. It's also not easy to say with certainty whether a patient will have a side effect or not.

Rheumatologists do try to make these assessments as they weigh up the history, the findings on examination, other health issues the patient may have and various test results.

For Rheumatoid Arthritis, "success" depends on many factors. Some of these include:

- the window of opportunity: earlier treatment leads to better outcomes;

- treating-to-target: use of medications & close monitoring of response with swapping of medications as needed to get a better response;

- poor prognostic factors: how aggressive the disease is, how many joints are affected, how much inflammation is present clinically or using imaging or blood tests;

- negative factors such as periodontal disease, smoking, excess weight, etc.

As a guide, Methotrexate works best early in the RA disease course with a good chance to achieve a remission state — around 40% using Methotrexate as the sole disease-modifying agent (DMARD).

This does not mean 60% do badly.

They will not have as good control of the disease and to obtain better control, changes or addition in medication therapy need to be considered.

**Rosiet:** "So, you would say that I, as newly diagnosed, have a decent chance for full remission considering the Plaquenil has given me some relief on its own. And, it is a matter of running through each drug to find a 'tolerance to healing' ratio? I will admit that after not being able to take the sulfasalazine and looking toward the MTX and its myriad of side effects I am feeling apprehensive, at best. Along the line of the 'tolerance to healing' ratio, in your opinion is there a gray area where side effects are accepted to a degree with good drug response?"

**My response:**

In general, Plaquenil would be considered a weak DMARD on its own. Most of us would start with Methotrexate as 1st line DMARD for Rheumatoid. I suppose there are occasions when rheumatologists would use Plaquenil at the start, for eg, if pregnancy was being pursued, or the prognosis of your type of Rheumatoid was considered very good (based on a range of features including those I listed previously).

There are of course gray areas.

Any treatment decision is a balance between the probability of a good result vs the possibility of a side effect.

Have you had similar worries to Rosiet you haven't voiced?

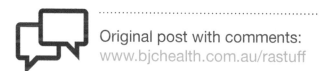

Original post with comments:
www.bjchealth.com.au/rastuff

One of the most common medications we use is corticosteroid. We often just refer to this as steroids. Prednisone or Predniso-lone is the most common form prescribed by rheumatologists.

In RA, this medication is often used at the start of treatment to get some rapid control of the inflammation. The conventional DMARDs take time to have an effect, usually weeks to months, so steroids play the part of a bridging therapy while we wait.

We're all very mindful of using steroids as this class of medication does have many side effects that occur commonly (unlike the possible side effects of the conventional DMARDs which occur much less commonly) when the steroids are used for a prolonged period as higher doses.

Use of corticosteroids is often debated and it causes angst among those who need it.

Some patients find it extremely hard to reduce their use of corticosteroids and I wanted to express that. Here are a few posts regarding this medication, which can be a two-edged sword.

## Dear Steroid, I love you...
Published August 11, 2013

Dear steroid (aka corticosteroid),

I have known you for so many years and I thought it was time to write to let you know my feelings.

I do love you. You've been there for me through thick and thin.

You really do good work. Most times, very quickly and so effectively reducing the pain and suffering for my arthritis patients. They often love you as well because you make their lives bearable.

At times, you are a lifesaver. Sometime, no other treatment works as quickly (think vasculitis or polymyalgia) and while you may need other medications to help you, you remain the rock for many a rheumatologist.

You've allowed me to use you in so many ways. You come in so many forms, so many doses, and can be delivered in so many different and reliable ways.

Nothing else comes close.

I'm sure you're going to continue to be part of my life.

## Dear Steroid, I hate you...
Published August 12, 2013

Dear steroid (aka corticosteroid),

When I first met you, I thought the world of you. Little did I know how you were going to turn out.

The side effects!

You've made me put on so much weight. My skin feels like paper and I keep bruising every time I bump something.

My blood pressure is high, there's sugar in my blood, you've hurt my eyes and you've made my muscles feel weak.

I hate the way I look. You've made my face puffy and look at my belly!

I've even heard that you'll go as far as making my bones crumble and break.

I hate you! I want you out of my life!

## Why Rheumatologists will continue to use steroid

Published August 13, 2013

I wrote the last two letters/posts to give you an idea of the love-hate relationship most rheumatologists have with this drug.

Now for a more balanced view.

When I use the term steroid, I mean corticosteroids (not anabolic steroids).

It is the most useful medication I have at my disposal. It gets my patients and me out of trouble. Quickly and efficiently. It is a crucial drug in some diseases and can be organ-saving and life-saving.

In some diseases, there is little other choice.

But, as rheumatologists we know of its potential side effects. Many of these are nasty and will almost certainly develop if large enough doses are used, for a prolonged period.

For a disease like rheumatoid arthritis & other inflammatory arthritis, it's why we prefer you to be on DMARD therapy. It's why we use different combinations to try and help reduce the reliance on steroid long term.

We do often still need to use the medication. But the rule of thumb is to use it at the *lowest dose possible to achieve the result we need, for the shortest time possible.*

It's important any reduction of steroid use be done in discussion with your rheumatologist. We don't want the disease to be destabilised and we don't want any ill effects from reducing the dose of steroid too quickly.

Please note that most of the comments above relate to oral corticosteroid. The other routes: topical, intravenous, intranasal, inhalation or injectable, have different side effect profiles.

It is regular use long term which is the biggest concern. Your rheumatologist will always try to use the lowest dose possible.

I know how patients react to steroids can be different.

Not just in how effective the drugs are or the possible side effects, but also in their cognitive response to this medication given the mixed messages they receive from friends and family trying to be helpful, the internet, and their various health professionals.

It's why a balanced discussion is needed right at the start.

What is your experience with this?


The most common biologic DMARDs used in RA worldwide are the TNF inhibitor medications. There was a lot of initial concern regarding potential longer term side effects with these potent immunosuppressive medications.

Long term databases to monitor people on these medications have now reached 15 years or so, and the major fears have been allayed.

This of course does not mean we should not be cautious with biologic DMARDs. The biggest risk remains that of increased and severe infections. However, the earlier use of these biologic agents, in people who are generally in better health has again meant that serious infections have affected the minority.

I always discuss risk of malignancy with my patients as it's a common worry. RA by itself increases the risk of skin cancers and lymphoma. With the use of biologic DMARDs, there has not been any clear increase in risk of lymphoma, leukaemia, or solid organ cancers such as breast or colon cancer.

There is a small but clear increased risk of skin cancers so surveillance is required.

While most attention tends to be paid to the serious but uncommon side effects, the most common side effect with the major TNF-inhibitors used in RA, is that of injection site reactions.

## What to do for that TNF-inhibitor injection site reaction?
Published September 22, 2014

An hour or so after her Enbrel injection, she noticed this rash. It steadily increased in size over the day. A little tender, a little itchy. She was otherwise well.

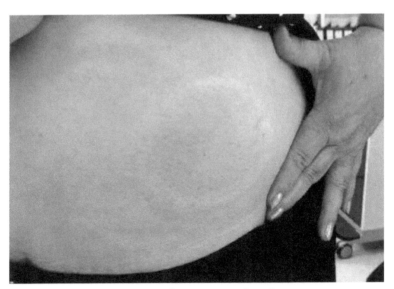

Injections site reactions do occur with subcutaneous injections, and they certainly do occur with the most commonly used biologic DMARDs, the TNF inhibitors.

What are our options?

- Do nothing if it's not particularly irritating for her. Most injection site reactions go away within a few days.

- Ice the area to reduce the swelling and to soothe the symptoms.

- Use an anti-histamine to reduce the swelling, itch and discomfort.

She should remember to rotate the sites of injection.

I've certainly had patients where the rash occurs with each injection. Sometimes, it's a very minor reaction. Less often, it's more pronounced as in this picture.

The 2 strategies I've used:

- Use an anti-histamine on the day of the injection, prior to the injection

- Swap the medication to another biologic DMARD. Injection site reactions are more common with Enbrel (Etanercept) and Humira (Adalimumab), and are less common with Simponi (Golimumab) and Cimzia (Certolizumab). Or we could swap to another class of biologic DMARD or swap to one with a different route of administration i.e. an Intravenous Infusion.

If you've had an injection site reaction, could you share with us how you managed it?

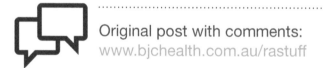

Original post with comments:
www.bjchealth.com.au/rastuff

As with all the medications discussed in this book, there is an important balancing act between the possible benefit and the possible side effects relevant to each person's individual situation and health state to be considered.

Detailed discussion regarding this needs to take place between patient and their treating rheumatology team.

# Chapter 8

## The Patient Experience

It's fair to say that I learned very little in university about what people experienced when they are given a diagnosis of a chronic, lifelong illness such as RA.

It's actually a big deal and yes, I have learnt a bit more as I listen to and treat more and more patients in my practice.

Two things helped me fast track my understanding.

Firstly, I've attended a number of appointments when my father was given a diagnosis of cancer. He's an intelligent man but the mix of apprehension, uncertainty, denial and despair, caused him to not ask any relevant questions, to not be able to recall what he was told, and to cope poorly in those first few months.

The oncology service was however fantastic with a designated coordinator who would touch base with him, set up the appointments he needed to attend, and provide a friendly face to negotiate the confusing medical system.

In rheumatology, with the complex autoimmune diseases we diagnose and manage, there is typically not this kind of support. I am sure most people are given handouts or told to find out a bit more on the internet, or worse still, they're just given the usual spiel in the clinic, leaving with a script for some medication that others will then warn them is dangerous.

Secondly, my time using social media, and particularly the interactions on my blog and on twitter, have exposed me to the different concerns and angst that those living with RA express.

It's strange that the rheumatology community often complains about the reduced adherence with our management plans if you follow the arguments above.

I do not have the answer to this issue as it will depend what resources the clinical service treating you has.

However, I feel more support at the time of diagnosis with as much, simple-to-understand education as is wanted, will help. I do not think all this can be done in the same consultation where the diagnosis is delivered.

People need time to digest the information, to come up with questions that matter to them, and to deal with their reactions or biases, and those of their families and friends. So the access to education and support needs to occur over time.

This can occur with clinic visits, with arthritis associations and other support groups, it can occur through using telecommunication eg email, telephone, or it can occur online.

I've written this book to provide some of the information needed.

There's of course a lot of help available online, in various formats. And it would be good if you learned from other people who have had to experience RA.

A few resources you could use as starting points are:

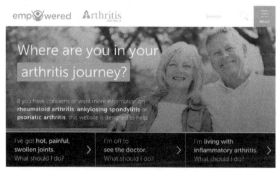

www.empowered.org.au

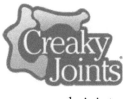

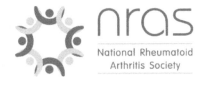

www.creakyjoints.org    www.nras.org.uk

A particular topic I need to mention is pregnancy. RA affects many decisions around this and it can be a very worrying and difficult process for both partners as they consider their options.

The following guest blog post is by Suzie Edward May, who has RA. I do recommend her book as it will highlight a number of complicated issues to help you in your discussions with your treating rheumatologist.

## Arthritis, pregnancy and the path to parenthood
Published October 2, 2013

**The following is a guest post by the author, Suzie Edward May:**

Pregnancy and babies are not usually something immediately associated with arthritis. While our community still holds ill-informed misconceptions about what arthritis is and whom it affects, issues like pregnancy and parenting for women (and men) with arthritis will remain out of people's minds. The reality is however (as you may well know), women living with chronic arthritis such as RA are having children everyday.

When my husband and I decided to start our family, I had lived with RA for 5 years. My illness had always been severe and I had grown dependent on a lot of medication to do the simplest daily tasks. Life was filled with constant pain, fatigue and uncertainty. When I spoke to my Rheumatologist about pregnancy, I was told I would need to come off all my medications over a period of months. This was a frightening prospect, as I had no idea what my body would be like without the crutch of medication. In fact, I had forgotten what it was like to live without pain everyday.

I searched worldwide for a resource that would explain to me how on earth I was meant to do this. I was desperate to speak with other women who had been through this process before me and succeeded. To my disbelief, I found nothing. I made a decision at that moment that I would document my journey and write a book about arthritis and pregnancy, to ensure other women did not feel the isolation and fear that I felt.

Through my research for the book, I found and connected with women all over the world who had been through this process before me. They all echoed the same message of isolation and lack of information but great inner strength. They inspired me to get through my own two challenging pregnancies and motivated me to publish my book, despite my own debilitating RA.

*Arthritis, pregnancy and the path to parenthood* was launched in March 2010 and has currently sold to women and men across 13 countries. It remains the only resource of its kind worldwide and has been endorsed by arthritis and consumer organizations globally. While it is written by a health consumer, primarily for health consumers, it is also relevant to family, friends and colleagues of people living with arthritis, as well as health and medical service providers.

Not only has the book filled a gap in information about arthritis and pregnancy, it has also started an important global discussion that recognizes the challenges faced by parents and future parents with arthritis. The book takes the reader on the journey from pre-conception to caring for their baby up to 12 months. It shares the very real experiences of women who have been through this process and helps to prepare the reader for the potential challenges that lay ahead.

I am proud of this book for a number of reasons. The main being that it is making a real difference in people's lives. So, while *Arthritis, pregnancy and the path to parenthood* remains relevant in its content, I will continue to seek and reach as many women and men as possible, so they don't feel alone.

Parenting is a magical gift and when you live with a chronic illness it can feel far out of reach. When you are in so much pain that even rolling over in bed or dressing yourself seems insurmountable, it can be very hard to imagine your body creating another life. But, with your medical team behind you and your loved ones alongside you, it is possible. I cherish my two children everyday and still find it incredible that my body, which has let me down in so many ways, created them.

*Arthritis, pregnancy and the path to parenthood*
is available at www.givingvoice.com.au

A good support network is invaluable.

The problem is the general lack of awareness of RA and what it entails. Many of the symptoms RA causes are not visible and people around those who have RA may not realise what they are experiencing.

Well-meaning friends and relatives may sometimes actually not be particularly helpful.

Many people with RA have been told that they just need to adjust their diet, or that they need to just take the latest fad supplement, or that they just need to see a particular chiropractor or naturo-path who was wonderful at fixing their friend's problem.

It's also unfortunate when friends and relatives disparage vari-ous medications and scare people with RA from taking appro-priate treatment.

Friends and relatives are of course trying to help but they may not understand the specifics of this disease.

I have however come into contact with many supportive spous-es, family members and caring friends.

By being empathic and by just being there to help, this support network can have a very positive impact on a patient's ability to self-manage and live a full life despite RA.

I also feel that a better understanding of the disease is likely to help the support network be more effective.

# Chapter 9

## Lifestyle change. Come on, take control!

Those with rheumatoid arthritis often enquire as to what else they can do to help with the disease control, apart from taking medications. I like it when this is raised and I think it is important that people take as much control as they can for their health.

Pain, stiffness, and fatigue typically lead to reduction in normal activities, and this in turn, can quickly lead to a degree of deconditioning. Muscles as well as ligaments and tendons, the structures around the joints, become weak.

In RA, there is also a higher risk of osteoporosis as inflammation leads to increased loss of bone density, and a higher incidence of cardiovascular disease, as inflammation promotes atherosclerosis. Atherosclerosis refers to the hardening of the arteries, as plaque builds up inside the arteries.

These can be helped with lifestyle modification.

Rheumatologists work with general practitioners to facilitate investigations including bone mineral density, blood tests for cholesterol, triglycerides and glucose. Problems such as hypertension and/or diabetes need to be optimally controlled.

For those who are overweight, weight loss will clearly make a difference. This requires attention to appropriate nutrition and portion/caloric control.

Exercise remains important (for all of us, with or without RA). Patients may be afraid of damaging their joints by exercising but this is unlikely to occur. Suitable low impact exercise is beneficial. During a flare with painful and swollen joints, it is not realistic to push yourself to exercise. Instead, the flare needs to be settled with medication, and exercise modified as required.

Dietary improvement and exercise should be co-prescribed with medication in RA. Doctors sometimes do not emphasise these enough and while we appreciate that lifestyle change is difficult to achieve, the overall benefits are clear.

There is also solid evidence that smoking increases the severity of rheumatoid arthritis, accelerates bone loss which may result in osteoporosis, and exponentially increases the risk of heart attacks and strokes.

Smoking cessation must be an integral part of rheumatoid arthritis treatment.

## Rheumatoid: you must stop smoking!
Published March 10, 2013

I was discussing rheumatoid arthritis management with a bunch of colleagues, and we were discussing various peculiarities and relative properties of the biologic medications.

At some stage, one rheumatologist mentioned that she finds herself spending more and more time addressing smoking cessation.

Patients with Rheumatoid Arthritis die from heart attacks and vascular complications.

This is well known, and the good news is that better disease control reduces the risk of this.

In addition, TNF inhibitor therapy reduces this risk of dying from cardiovascular causes more than the traditional DMARDs.

But we can do more. Weight loss and improved nutrition, increased exercise to improve fitness, treating blood pressure, et cetera.

Often, the hardest nut to crack is SMOKING.

Smoking is not good for Rheumatoid because:

- It acts as a trigger leading to the disease

- It leads to more active disease

- It reduces the effectiveness of Methotrexate

- It reduces the effectiveness of TNF-inhibitor therapy

And by the way, if you didn't already know, smoking does cause lung damage, increases risk of cancer, and greatly increases the risk of strokes and heart attacks.

I remarked to this very caring and competent rheumatologist that I wasn't very good at getting my patients to stop smoking.

If you're a smoker, what can I say to you to make you stop? Because, you really do need to.

There are rows and rows of supplements in most pharmacies with many benefits being claimed. So, it's not a surprise that many people purchase these supplements to try and help their RA.

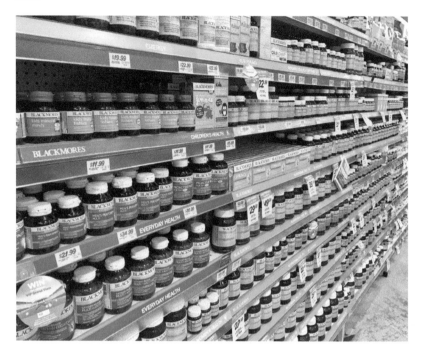

There is however little evidence to suggest any benefit in RA for the bulk of these. This includes glucosamine with or without chondroitin.

The one supplement which does help treat RA is fish oil. The following blog post from my colleague, Dr Rob Russo, will address this.

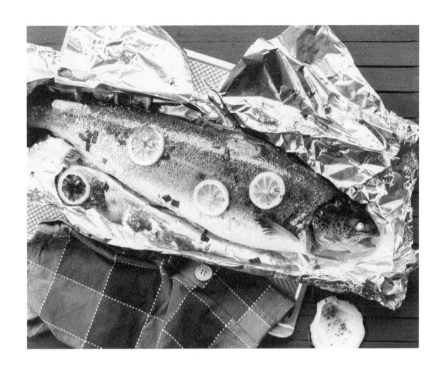

## Fish Oil, will you now use this for RA?
Published November 18, 2013

By Dr Roberto Russo, Rheumatologist

Fish oil has literally become the flavour of the month!

So much so that there are now a host of variants available on the shelf, including Super Fish oil, liquid fish oil, and Krill oil, with each option promising an advantage over the other! The popularity of the product seems to be ever increasing, particularly in the management of cardiovascular disease and joint conditions. The latter is the primary focus of this article.

The beneficial constituents of Fish oil are the omega-3 fatty acids, **eicosapentaenoic acid (EPA) and docosahexanoic**

**acid (DHA)**. These have been shown to suppress inflammatory mediators including:

- Proinflammatory lipid mediators
- Prostaglandin E2
- Leukotriene B4
- Peptide mediators
- TNF-alpha
- IL-1 beta

These are effectively the same inflammatory mediators that are inhibited by the use of NSAIDs and the biological TNF blockers (albeit at a much lesser extent), thereby providing a biological plausibility to their use (especially in inflammatory joint conditions)!

However, the amount of EPA+DHA required to obtain symptomatic benefit in this context is relatively high at greater than **2.7 g each day**, which is more than is required for cardiovascular benefit.

The standard Fish oil capsule contains about 400 mg of EPA+DHA and as such a patient would need to take at least 7 of those capsules a day, which would challenge even the most ardent of patients to comply with such a regime! No wonder there are so many options available (as mentioned above).

But does Fish oil have a real benefit in patients with Rheumatoid arthritis, especially in the context of the modern management of the disease, which often involves the use of a combination of immunomodulating drugs to render the disease into remission?

That is the exact question that a group of our colleagues from South Australia set out to answer.

They chose to divide a cohort of patients with early Rheumatoid arthritis (defined as <12 months) into two groups, whereby one received 10mL of liquid Fish oil (providing

5.5g/day) and the other a low dose equivalent to 400mg/day, which is the dose often taken for cardiovascular disease.

Both groups were then treated for their disease according to the current standard approach, whereby disease modifying medications (DMARDs) were introduced in sequential order (including TNF blockers if required), with the aim being to achieve remission (a strategy termed treat to target).

What they found was the group receiving a high dose of Fish oil:

- Required a shorter time to achieve a meaningful improvement in their disease control

- Achieved a higher the rate of remission (according to the American College of Rheumatology criteria)

- Had a lower failure rate to triple DMARD therapy, thereby requiring less use of TNF blockers

- Required less use of NSAIDs

No differences though were found in overall disease activity, dose of Methotrexate or Prednisone used, or physical function.

The concern for an increased risk of bleeding was not found in their study, albeit I would remain cautious in prescribing Fish oil in those on blood thinning medications such as Warfarin or a combination of anti-platelet agents.

In conclusion, it would appear that there are indeed benefits to be gained with the use of high dose Fish oil as an adjunct to the current approach of treating Rheumatoid arthritis.

I would encourage you to read the article in full, which can be found in the Annals of Rheumatic Diseases (reference given below).

Whilst I am already in the habit of suggesting my patients take Fish oil, these results strengthen my conviction in this recommendation and remind me to ensure they are taking a sufficient amount.

I look forward to reading similar high quality research regarding the use of Fish oil in other joint diseases, especially in Osteoarthritis.

If you are a doctor, I would be most interested to know if you recommend fish oil, and if so what doses to you suggest?

If you are a patient, have you been recommended fish oil, and if so what doses do you take?

*Reference: Proudman SM, James MJ, et al. Fish oil in recent onset Rheumatoid arthritis: a randomised, double-blind controlled trial within algorithm-based drug use. Annals of Rheumatic Disease, 2013; 0: 1-7. doi:10.1136/annrheumdis-2013-204145*

While I am happy for my patients with RA to try supplements, I do suggest that it would be better to attend to improving their diet (as well as stopping smoking and finding time for regular exercise).

It's hard for most doctors to provide detailed, useful, practical advice and it's harder still for patients to just search the net for this advice given what is on the internet can often be quite contradictory when it comes to anti-inflammatory eating for arthritis and autoimmune disease.

So, it's important to try and make things easier, using whole foods that are fresh and seasonal, and which can be easily sourced.

The dietitians at my clinic have worked hard on a cookbook resource, making it relevant and as balanced as possible using a blend of experience and the literature.

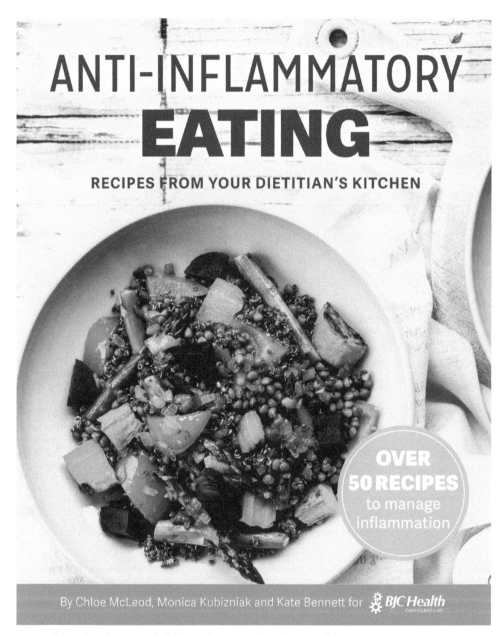

**ANTI-INFLAMMATORY EATING**

RECIPES FROM YOUR DIETITIAN'S KITCHEN

OVER
50 RECIPES
to manage
inflammation

By Chloe McLeod, Monica Kubizniak and Kate Bennett for **BJC Health**
connected care

This book is available at: https://shop.bjchealth.com.au

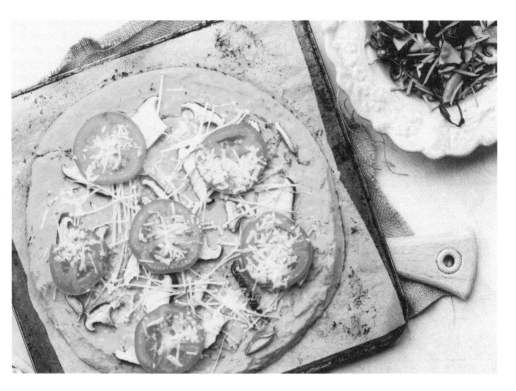

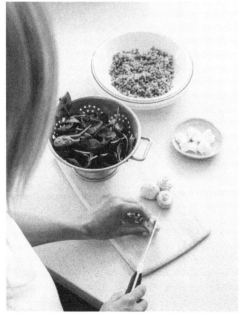

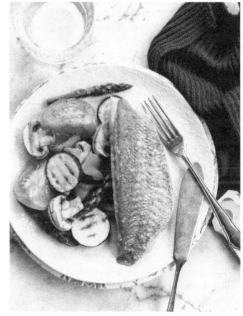

Having a chronic illness may lead to a degree of anxiety and stress. It makes life more difficult to deal with.

In turn, the difficulties and stresses of daily life can make RA more difficult to deal with, and some people find that periods of heightened stress flare their disease.

It's often difficult to help people manage this aspect of RA.

Altering job hours or the nature of the work could be useful. Timetabling sessions for relaxation and exercise may help. Mindfulness exercises are used by some.

Occasionally, counselling is required. Sometimes, it's helpful to just be aware of this aspect of disease self-management and to attempt to reduce life stressors as much as possible.

# Chapter 10

## The C Word

I can't cure RA but here's what we'll achieve

Published September 27, 2015

It's Sunday just after 6am. Wet and cold outside. The house is quiet and it's a great time to write.

I'm preparing a talk on rheumatoid arthritis and as I read through some source material, I'm contemplating how far we've come in improving the management of this disease. There's still however a range of unmet needs or wants.

I think I know what my patients with rheumatoid want.

**Cure.**

I can't deliver that. No rheumatologist can.

But we can and will clearly improve treatment. Here's a wish list:

- To be able to achieve remission & sustain this remission in a higher percentage of patients.

- To get the vast majority of patients into a low disease activity state.

- In those who've achieved prolonged remission, to be able to discontinue the medication without a flare or return of disease.

- To completely prevent damage and deformity.

- To reduce the potential side effects of the medication we use. We want safer & safer options.

- To be able to individualise patient therapy. We would love to be able to confidently pick the very best treatment for each patient.

The goalposts have clearly changed. Things have improved for patients with rheumatoid arthritis and for the rheumatologists who treat this condition.

While I know that list is missing the "C" word, I hope you can take some comfort in the improvements to come. Please feel free to share your thoughts.

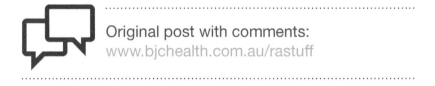

Original post with comments:
www.bjchealth.com.au/rastuff

# Chapter 11

## Concluding Thoughts

If you've read through the book to this page, you already know more about RA than many health professionals.

That's a good thing.

I do believe that educating yourself equips you to better deal with this disease.

Especially when the disease is confusing and you may be scared about the future, and very hesitant about the use of medications.

This is not meant to be an authoritative text on RA so please accept my apologies if I've missed out on discussing some aspect that you are particularly interested in. I've definitely not been able to cover every symptom and presentation or detail every medication or strategy. I have not attempted to explain the interplay between genetics, the environment and the interactions between the various parts of our immune system as I do not believe I have sufficient expertise to make this easy to understand.

I have however attempted to craft a resource which is accessible to you and your loved ones.

My hope is that this will allow you to contribute to and understand shared decisions regarding your health.

Engage with your health and establish an open and honest partnership with a team of healthcare professionals you can trust. It will make things easier.

Feel free to contact me. I'd love you to share your thoughts.

*Irwin Lim*

@_connectedcare

www.bjchealth.com.au/bjc-blogs

*Here are links to other resources which we think will be useful:*

Rheumatoid Arthritis Xplained: an illustrated flip-through story
www.raxplained.com.au/ra-app-page

Our Youtube channel, containing a range of content, including stuff on RA www.youtube.com/user/bjchealthAU/playlists

Our Facebook page where you can interact with our team of professionals www.facebook.com/BJCHealth.ConnectedCare

The Empowered website: more detailed videos including stories of people living with inflammatory arthritis
www.empowered.org.au

*Arthritis, pregnancy and the path to parenthood*: a great book on this difficult subject www.givingvoice.com.au/book

*Anti-Inflammatory Eating: Recipes from Your Dietitian's Kitchen*
www.bjchealth.com.au/anti-inflammatory-cookbook

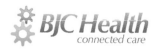